I'll Shave My Head Too

A Father's Stories Through the Happy Hell of Childhood Cancer

by Steve Dolling

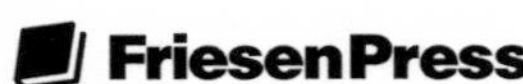

Suite 300 - 990 Fort St
Victoria, BC, Canada, V8V 3K2
www.friesenpress.com

First Edition — 2015

Edited by Krissy Darch and Rob Kragelj
With stories by Spencer Dolling
www.shavemyheadtoo.com

ISBN
978-1-4602-6115-6 (Hardcover)
978-1-4602-6116-3 (Paperback)
978-1-4602-6117-0 (eBook)

1. Health & Fitness, Diseases, Cancer

Distributed to the trade by The Ingram Book Company

For Tracey

My love who perpetuates the outrageous

lie helping us all live truthfully.

Induction

In-duc-tion: 1) the first line treatment for cancer, usually involving high doses of chemotherapy 2) that period of time when the child accepts having no hair, and the parent accepts the loss of their mind 3) the stories of Spencer from age six to age eight

The Outrageous Lie

Spencer was six years old. Nearly seven. He wasn't well. He was pale and losing weight. He was listless and had fevers that wouldn't go away. His "flu" seemed to be dragging on.

Tracey had taken him to the doctor several times without result. Finally, she called the doctor at home one Saturday morning with renewed concern and he more or less told her that she was being an overreactive worrying fuss of a mother. Tracey is not the over-reacting type. She hung up and took Spencer to the local walk-in clinic while I took Foster, our youngest son, down to the boat to go fishing with his cousins.

Tracey called from the local clinic where the doctor had found a lump in Spencer's abdomen that he didn't like. He wanted to send Spencer for an X-ray, so within a few hours of the first call to the doctor, I was on my way to meet Tracey and Spencer at the local hospital.

The ER docs at the local hospital showed us a picture of a suspicious mass. Someone used the word *'oncologist'*. They suggested we get a notebook to write down our questions so we would remember them. Within a few hours of the X-ray, we were on our way to Children's Hospital.

At Children's, there were a million health history questions. A medical student seemed particularly interested in whether Spencer had been exposed to bear feces. We held out hope that maybe Spencer had been playing in the woods and unknowingly exposed himself to toxic bear poop.

Three days later, after what seemed like dozens of tests, we sat down for The Meeting. All hope of bear shit disease was dispelled. One doctor took our notebook and started writing notes for us while we sat in silence, learning from the other doctor about stage IV neuroblastoma.

Spencer had a tumour the size of a grapefruit wrapped around his adrenal gland. The disease had metastasized to various bones in his body, including his pelvis and skull. Untreated, it would all be over very quickly.

He would need chemotherapy to shrink the tumour, surgery to remove it, possibly radiation to the tumour bed followed by more chemotherapy. Then there was something that sounded like a bone marrow transplant, but they called a "stem cell" transplant. He would finish up with some other treatment called retinoic acid — a drug they use for severe acne in adolescents.

They were going to cure our kid with pimple cream.

This was the worldwide, best practice treatment protocol for stage IV neuroblastoma. Total duration of treatment: about six months. Chance of long-term survival: about 25%.

Any questions?

Forget about pimple creams for Spencer the teenager; he was going to need luck to survive second grade. Neuroblastoma is not one of the gentler cancers. It doesn't have the 80% cure rates of some of the other kid's ones. There is very little research and there are no pink ribbons. It's a killer without a cause.

I sat in bed with him that night in the hospital watching TV and explained that we were going to move to another ward. A lot of the kids there would be bald. They would have no hair.

"Why are they bald?" Spencer asked.

I explained. "They take very powerful medicine for their cancer and it makes their hair fall out."

Spencer asked, "Will my hair fall out?"

"Yes."

"Oh," he said.

"Would you like it if I shaved my head and was bald too?" I asked.

"Yes, that would be good." And that was that. Just a matter-of-fact acceptance and he moved forward, wondering what was on the other TV channels.

That moment, for me, was the beginning of the outrageous lie. Kids have no hang-ups or preconceived notions about the stuff that terrifies adults. They don't suffer based on notions of what the future might be. They live here and now and maybe tomorrow. They have no reason to believe something ought to be terrifying unless it looks scary, makes a loud noise, or causes them pain.

Or it scares the adults.

They take their cues from us, so we need to be positive and optimistic.

That happy optimism is the outrageous lie, the impossible parenting skill.

It is the smile I put on my face as we watched TV. The hospital room birthday party for Tracey. The detour we take on the way home to pick up a Nintendo GameCube as we worry about the new bumps forming on his head. The plans we make for playing games as we check into the hospital for chemo a few days later. The coloured dye in my hair before the shaving. The electric go kart engineered by the uncles. The smiles, the good news, and the reports for the friends and relatives.

After a bit, the lie becomes so fully embraced and internalized that it's utterly indistinguishable from the truth.

We are happy. We are optimistic. The first round of chemo brought near instant relief. The bumps disappeared. My, how good Spencer looks bald! Hospital life isn't so bad, and Spencer goes to school between treatments. Look how quickly he recovered from surgery! We are going to beat this thing and have fun doing it, damn it!

It was the truth. There was more laughter than there were tears. Spencer lived to see third grade! And fourth. And the others. And he became a teenager, with remarkably flawless skin.

Tracey became an expert on neuroblastoma. She would share the latest research with the team. Together with the doctors, we figured out what comes after acne treatments. Good news was good. Bad news just needed a new plan.

We felt a little sad for the other families. The ones with the healthy kids who weren't living life as fully as they could.

Somewhere along the way, I began to write these stories. They spilled out of my brain and on to the keyboard because there just isn't enough room inside for the outrageous lie and the truth to reside together. The stories were my way of surviving.

The stories are outrageous lies. Every word is true.

A Dark Night on 3B

Since the time of Spencer's diagnosis, there hasn't been any really bad news. From the outset, we expected a journey with ups and downs — positive progress and setbacks along the way. But really, it's all been good, so far. Until now.

Sure, there has been a scare or two. There was a bone scan that Tracey saw that had her pretty much convinced that the cancer was spreading rapidly. She took the kids for passport photos hoping we would have a chance to squeeze in Disneyland. As it turned out, the contrast was just set a little differently in the machine. The doctors were pleased with the scan, as they pointed out to us a few days later.

There was round three of chemo — that nasty event that henceforth became known as "The Vomit Festival". Truly unpleasant, but nasty as it was, we knew it was just part of the treatment. The 15% of his body weight that he lost came back in just a few short weeks.

There was that one summary I did where I itemized all the tests, pokes, and treatments that Spencer had undergone in a month. It was truly alarming. The numbers have since doubled, tripled or gone up ten times, but they are all just steps on the path.

Last night was different. I should have known it was coming, but somehow we've avoided it all this time.

The ominous signs were there earlier in the day. Spencer's roommate, an eleven-year-old boy, was having a difficult afternoon. He just wanted to stop his chemotherapy and go home. I don't blame him. At some point, you just get fed up. You can bet his mom was having an equally tough day.

Elsewhere in the ward, things were much worse. Tracey told us that they asked for the hallways to be cleared for a "private transfer". A brave kid that didn't make it all the way to a cure.

All the signs were bad.

It happened at 12:20 am. It wasn't Spencer's nurse who came. They sent the most experienced nurse — the leader on the ward — the one who has dealt with all the toughest situations with grace and dignity. This was to be one of her rougher assignments.

She woke me with a smile. The smile was meaningless. That is not to say it wasn't genuine or had a ring of insincerity. No. The smile is just part of her professional uniform. It reflects something deep in the character of an oncology nurse that allows them to help people through the most difficult time in their lives. It is genuine and sincere. But you know that with the smile and professionalism can come words that can unglue your very soul.

The oncology parent is a different breed as well. We, too, are professionals. We deal with the meanest, roughest stuff that life can possibly throw at us and do it with grace and style. We check our kids into hospitals with life threatening infections and our major concern is that we might be too late to fill out the menu for the next day's meal choices.

I am one of those oncology parents. I can be woken from a deep sleep, see the smile, and be mentally prepared in an instant for what follows. My reaction will not be one of shock or horror. The words can slip through my mind and then rip through my gut, but I won't come unglued — at least visibly.

The words came, but there was something a little strange about the delivery. They came with a bit of a giggle, almost, but not quite, a violation of that professional code that exists between parents and oncology nurses. "Your snoring… It's so loud that she can't sleep," she said, nodding to the mother on the other side of the room. "Do you think you could sleep in the playroom? We'll come and get you if Spencer wakes up."

Bone Scan

Today is Tuesday, so it must be bone scan day. This is a routine test, but with the potential for outcomes that are anything but routine, we don't treat it lightly. Then there was the second bone scan. That's the one I treated as routine. I came home that night and Tracey had already taken the boys for passport photos because it looked like things were bad. Disney World would be a rush job. Two days later, we found out everything was okay. It was a wakeup call.

From then on, we had two new rules: 1) Whenever there is a test, hope for the best, but be prepared for the worst — nothing is routine. 2) Amateur radiology is a highly entertaining sport, but in our family, it must be practiced with great care.

Spencer was injected with the preferred isotope of whatever at nine this morning. I joined them at the hospital around 11:00 am for the scan. The scanner is a truly impressive machine. Children's Hospital was the first in Canada to take delivery of this particular model with the built-in DVD player. Spencer was strapped onto a rolling table while two large passive detection arrays slowly worked their way down his body, following the terrain like cruise missiles in slow motion. When his head emerged, he was able to watch the day's preferred video selection — Spiderman.

Now, knowing that amateur radiology is not something we should engage in, we couldn't help but let our attention drift from the movie to the display screens over at the operator's console. We could tell that things were looking pretty good. No return of those nasty spots on the side of his skull. Nothing glowing bright but the joint areas where new bone mimics neuroblastoma. Nothing to worry about.

Then a few bright spots emerge. The bladder full of isotope of whatchamacallit shines bright. No worries.

And then it came.

It was obvious even to us amateurs. At least one, maybe both testicles looked fully involved. It would be a few days before word got back from the radiologist through the oncologist with the real story, but in the meantime, we just sucked it in and waited for the news.

The scan was finished and the tech approached us. She wanted to do one more scan. Of course. She could see it too. The radiologist is going to want to have a closer look at the affected area. So much for routine.

She gave me a hospital gown and asked me to take Spencer to get changed. I hadn't seen him in a hospital gown in a long time. It's not a comfortable feeling. A little depressing, frankly.

We came back and remounted the machine. Somehow, Spiderman seemed more intensely enjoyable rather than irrelevant. I'm not sure why. It was kind of surreal.

The scan progressed. The tech confirmed what she suspected: radioactive urine dribbles in the underwear.

Nothing that can't be fixed with a load of laundry!

Nagging Question

Since diagnosis, the changes for Spencer have been quite dramatic. He couldn't go through six rounds of chemotherapy, a stem cell transplant, major surgery and six months in and out of the hospital without it having a profound effect. He is a lot tougher and has aged well beyond those six months. Nevertheless, he is still very much the wonderful boy he was when this all started.

Now for me, the changes have been a little more subtle. Okay, well, some not so subtle. The coloured Mohawk, for example, perhaps indicated a sudden and dramatic shift, but it quickly gave way to a more socially acceptable sheen sported by a broad cross section of society with or without overactive testosterone.

Since I was messing with the hair, the little goatee and moustache seemed like a fine addition. Piercings were a fairly natural follow-on contemplation, though I could never quite decide on which ones to get. My sister Vicki's suggestion that I just get them "all" seemed like a good idea, but once I discovered what "all" truly entailed, fear of pain won out over curiosity.

Then there was the whole weight thing. Spencer would have a round of chemotherapy. He would shed a few kilos. The family diet would adjust so that just about everything included a cup of whipped cream. He would put on a few kilos, and I would follow suit. He would have another round and lose a few kilos, but I wouldn't. Another fat-filled frolic and he puts on a few kilos; I put on a few kilos, and on it goes. The ratchet effect has left me at an all-time high for body mass.

The next bit is a little sensitive, but would really be obvious to anyone who cared to think about it. You see, the only time Tracey and I see each other anymore is when we change shifts at the hospital. There really aren't any private moments, if you know what I mean.

But she is a sweetheart. Just the other day, she was thinking of me and brought me back some slip-on shoes. They're the perfect thing for when you're up ten times a night in the hospital and you can't touch the floor. My immediate reaction was, "These are girlie shoes. I can't wear girlie shoes!" And then I tried them on. It turns out, they are the most comfortable shoes I've ever had. I love them.

So none of these things are terribly alarming individually. Collectively though, they're a little scary. You've got a man drifting into middle age who starts shaving his head bald, grows a beard, puts on twenty pounds, starts wearing women's shoes, and stops having sex with his wife. What does it all add up to? That's right. Sounds like a classic case when you view it all with an objective sense of detachment.

Late onset homosexuality.

Now don't get me wrong. I have no attraction to men, but I'm starting to get a little concerned. There's this guy who runs the coffee shop downstairs: Bald head, little beard and moustache. Has a voice that runs an octave above normal. I have an idea what his sexual orientation might be. I'm not being judgmental; he seems like a wonderful person. Lately he's been smiling and laughing a lot when I come around. In the past week he's given me two free cups of coffee. I thought it was just because I'm such a good customer, but now I'm starting to wonder.

I'm generally confident in my sense of self and particularly my own sexuality, but I find I now have this nagging question. If I can take a detached look at myself, connect the dots, and draw the obvious (though erroneous) conclusion, what are other people thinking?

Informed Consent

This isn't one of those stories with a bit of drama followed by a quirky twist that tickles the funny bone. I have to advise you of the risk before we begin. It's your choice whether you care to read on. Fair warning.

Informed consent. It's the foundation of all the non-emergency treatment and diagnostic procedures that they do at the hospital. Whether it was created as the outcome of some enlightened medical care philosophy or thrust into the healthcare realm by an overly zealous legal system doesn't really matter. Inherently, you have the right to choose. Nobody can do anything to your child without your okay. The decisions are yours.

So how does it all start for the typical cancer family? Some hideous sequence of events brings you to Children's Hospital. The first things they need to do are tests. Lots and lots of tests. "Yes, we would like to do an ultrasound, X-ray, CT scan, bone scan, more blood tests, and an MIBG to accurately diagnose and stage your child's disease." Yes, you get to choose whether to subject your child.

What inevitably follows is some definitive diagnosis and a treatment protocol. The reams of chemotherapeutic agents all have side effects. "This one causes baldness, that one causes high frequency hearing loss, this one can affect the kidneys, that one can affect the heart, nausea is a common side effect, etc." You listen with a sense of bewilderment and some amusement. You have a choice but don't even bother to ask about the alternative. You already knew the first time you heard them say the word "cancer".

Depending on what you're up against, surgery might be part of the game. A general anesthesia alone sounds like a bad risk. Once the surgeons fully detail all the potential complications of what might happen when your kid's particular tumour is removed, you sometimes wonder about the benefit of being informed. It doesn't leave you with a sense of comfort, but at least you have the choice.

Then there is the bone marrow or stem cell transplant. Now that meeting is a happy one. Let's contemplate the potential major organ failures: kidney, liver, lungs, bone marrow, and very occasionally, the heart. "Oh, and there is some risk to the brain, but generally not unless the other organs go first. Oh yes, and of course there is the chance of infection. Your options are bacterial, fungal and viral. They are all potentially lethal, but we do our best." Strangely enough, they don't even mention hair loss as an adverse side effect on this one. Remind me again of the options, please, I have a choice to make.

These are the impossible choices. Not that it is impossible to choose one way or the other. It just feels impossible to believe you are in the situation to begin with. Impossible to believe that you might eventually reach a point where you might want to consider option B.

But it's not all high-drama. Every day there are a bunch of informed medical decisions to be made. "Would he like this medicine in liquid form or can he take a pill? Gravol now or should we wait and try to space it between the Ondansetron doses? Platelets are low today, but not real low, we could hold off until tomorrow to transfuse if you can come back to the clinic. He's losing weight; we should consider an NG tube." And on and on and on.

These are all the meaningless choices, but not meaningless in the sense that they are unimportant. Do a good job on all the day-to-day stuff and it can have a big impact on your child's comfort and your peace of mind. Make all the wrong choices, though, and it won't likely have any effect on the final outcome. In that sense, they're all meaningless.

With all the impossible and meaningless choices that you get to make, is control just an illusion? Isn't it just one great train ride you are on, and at some point you pass a switch in the track that determines your final destination?

That might be true, but there is another choice you get to make that does have a lot of meaning. It may or may not affect the destination, but it certainly does affect the ride. It's not even an obvious choice because nobody will ever present it to you. You don't have to sign the consent form. You don't even have to announce your decision.

You get to choose how miserable you want to be.

Okay, life sucks. Your kid has cancer. But every day you get to choose if you want to be pessimistic or optimistic. You get to choose whether you want to be a victim or your kid's biggest champion. You get to choose if you want to endure the day or have some fun and make the best of it whatever it brings you. You get to choose what example you want to set for your kid. And you get to choose whether you want to teach your kid that he has a choice of whether to be miserable. It's a choice that you get to make a dozen times a day in different circumstances.

Once you realize that you have control over just about everything in your life, except perhaps the impossible choices and impossible outcomes, it makes the journey a whole lot easier. You might still be lumbering down the railroad, but if you believe you're flying the space shuttle, you might have a better chance of reaching escape velocity. And it's a whole lot more fun to eat astronaut food.

Disturbed Child

People always ask how Spencer's brother Foster is coping. The truth is, there are signs of stress. He's had a lot of separation from Mom and Dad. On a good day, he gets an hour with one or the other of us, seldom both. Over time, it is starting to have an impact.

We notice subtle things in behaviour. For example, his eating habits continue to diverge from the normal four-year-old diet. The other night I came home and our friend Donna said that Foster didn't touch the chicken fingers and fries that were served for dinner. He did, however have three platefuls of sushi — enough for an adult. Is this normal for a four-year-old? I don't know. Sometimes people tell me he didn't eat much for dinner. Sometimes they can't believe how much food he can pack in. Sometimes he has a cookie for a bedtime snack. Sometimes he likes green olives and a couple of crab sticks.

But hey, that's just diet. It doesn't indicate your kid has any problems — maybe just sophisticated tastes. I can live with that. But there are other, more disturbing signs. For quite a while we would put him to bed all nicely dressed up in his pajamas. We would go to check on him in the middle of the night and he would be buck-naked. He would come down in the morning with his pajamas on again. His explanation: "I just like to sleep like Dad does." Now that's disturbing. The trend does seem to have eased now that fall weather is here. Maybe he just has a sophisticated sense of thermal control.

Ah, but there are other cracks. Real signs that deep trouble is lurking under the mop of blonde hair. Take, for instance, his unnatural fascination with his Uncle John. It's probably due to too much separation from Dad. John has become the reference standard against which all things are measured: "Daddy, who's bigger: That kid or Uncle Johnny?" "Daddy, who's larger: Your truck or Uncle Johnny? Is Uncle Johnny bigger than Canada?"

Then at night as I tuck him into bed, "Daddy, who's stronger: You or Uncle Johnny?" Uh oh. This one needs a careful answer. Better not fumble it or it could have lasting implications. Johnny has about a 3-inch height advantage and though we may have roughly the same displacement, let's just say that he has a higher density distribution.

"Well, Foster… Uncle Johnny is a pretty big guy, but Daddy is mean and tough." There, that ought to do it. No lies. No lifelong hang-ups about the inadequacy of his father.

"Daddy, I think Uncle Johnny is stronger."

"Oh, and why would you think that, Foster?"

"Because he's an engineer."

So all that is just a sign that he is well-bonded with his uncle. Nothing to worry about. Well, here's one that convinces me it's about time to bring Spencer home and get the family life back to normal. Tracey put Foster to bed last night. A little while later, she walked into the room. She heard him muttering away. On closer examination, it seemed as though he was playing with his stuffed animals.

"Girl… Girl… Girl…" He was picking each one up, turning it over and doing a thorough inspection. "Girl... Girl..."

"What are you doing, Foster?"

"Just checking, Mom. They're all girls."

Not a penis to be found on any of his teddy bears.

To Whom It May Concern:

I don't want to strike a lot of controversy, or carry on a dialogue that's not appropriate for this forum. Let's just say that You and I have never talked before, and there are a few things I would like to get off my chest. Obviously, this is a bit of strange way to reach You, but there are some really thoughtful people here with closer connections than me who might be able to pass along the message if it doesn't get there by a more direct route. Let's be frank: I don't know where "there" is or exactly who You are, but I think the things I want to say may be relevant in any case.

First of all, I have to say I'm a little bit upset about this whole neuroblastoma thing. There has been a lot of suffering, pain and misery. It's a horrible thing to subject a child to, and it's really not pleasant for the rest of the family. The fear and anxiety are ever-present. I would have much rather had my heart ripped out than have this happen to Spencer. I don't think it really matters whether You had any direct involvement, it happened on Your watch, and I am angry about that.

Enough said. Now for the more important stuff. There are a few things for which I am extremely grateful. Things that in the everyday course of life, I didn't think enough about or have a deep enough appreciation for.

Many mornings now, I wake up and see my boys sleeping peacefully and think it's a glorious day just because they are alive and here. Thanks.

The strength, caring, and love of Tracey are profound beyond words. For that, I am hugely appreciative. Thanks.

I don't really care if the grass gets mowed, or the meeting gets attended, or the car gets washed. It's a whole lot easier to select the little things that, when added together, are important in the grand scheme and not sweat stuff that really doesn't matter. And careers, money, nice cars and the like now rank among the small stuff for me. Thanks.

I enjoy it sometimes when the boys argue, carry on, or get excessively silly. It's a wonderful thing to have them so full of life and vitality. I have to work harder to get annoyed. Thanks.

I can listen to someone pour their heart out about the miseries and pains of everyday life, feel for them and have comforting words, but not be at all alarmed knowing what incredible capacity ordinary people have to cope with everyday misfortune. Thanks.

Friends and family have an amazing capacity for love, caring and concern that you just don't see or appreciate every day. I do now. Thanks.

When life is at its most tumultuous and extreme, somehow it's possible to gain a new sense of perspective, which puts you in a better balance than you ever had before. Bizarre. Thanks.

And finally, thank you for giving me the voice to talk about things like this, that I never would have talked about before. I feel better now. If You are there and listening, we would sure appreciate a good outcome for Spencer.

The Monster

There's a monster. It lives in our house.

It moved in a long time ago. It must have been hiding in the walls because we didn't notice it for the longest time. But it was there. It's the funniest thing, because I never really believed in monsters. I thought they were the stuff of fairy tales. Imaginary beasts that people made up to explain their fears. They weren't real though. Were they?

Now I know they are. The thing about monsters is that they're not just big and scary with sharp teeth. Bears are big and scary with sharp teeth, but they're not monsters. The difference is that the monster has a malevolent streak. It's not there because it wants to eat your garbage; it's there because it means to do you harm. Disney got it all wrong in *Monsters, Inc.* Don't believe it. That's all imaginary. Those kinds of cute cuddly monsters don't exist. Stephen King has it right.

The monster sometimes comes into our room at night and slithers underneath the bed. Its hot breath comes right through the mattress. It leaves me sweating, scared and unable to sleep. And then a chill settles in like the window was left open on a January night.

We've tried to kill it a dozen times. Sometimes it seems like we're winning, but still it won't die. Even if we kill it, I have this terrible feeling it will come back from the dead like in the sequel to a bad horror movie.

It's a clever beast and follows us wherever we go. There's no escape. We can never see it because it hides in the shadows, but it's always there and has ways of making its presence known. We can't live a normal life.

When we got the dog, we thought maybe he would scare the monster away. The dog is smart and brave, but somehow he doesn't see the monster. The monster, though, is keeping its distance. But somehow I think it might be smarter than the dog and just waiting for its moment. Try to explain a monster to your friends. They can hear what we're saying, but they don't quite believe us. We still have all of our body parts, and none of us has quite gone insane. They've never seen the monster, even though they've been to the house. Still they get the sense that something isn't quite right. Some of them keep their distance. Now we just smile and say, "Oh the monster... he's gone back inside the wall. We're doing fine."

Sometimes our monster doesn't seem so scary. On a sunny day, when the kids run in the park laughing and playing, we forget that it's back there waiting for us. You have to forget for a while, or it will get inside your mind and drive you over the edge.

There are professionals who know how to deal with monsters. Ordinary folks never meet them, other than on a social basis. We feel better when we're with the professionals. They seem to know what they're doing. But at night when we are home alone, there's just us... and the monster. The chill returns.

There's a monster. It lives in our house. It lives in our boy.

Essential Tools

Spencer came home with a nasal gastric tube. An NG tube is a small hose that goes down through the nose and into the stomach. He'll likely get a good portion of his daily caloric intake this way for the next week or two. After the first time, the horror and degree of discomfort anticipated by a seven-year-old boy contemplating having the next one stuffed up his nose and down his throat are indescribable.

So there we were last night. Spencer had a nice meal of KFC. He's feeling great. After dinner he wants to try on Halloween costumes — he's planning on being Harry Potter. That's all very nice because we didn't really even expect him to be out of the hospital in time for Halloween.

Now there's a small problem. Harry Potter isn't bald, but that's okay because Nanny bought this crazy wig for just this purpose. So on goes the costume — but you can't have Harry Potter with hair down to his shoulders. No, you have to trim the wig. Cut it down to size. So off Spencer and Mom go into the bathroom to cut the wig. You already know where this is going, don't you?

Yes, that's right. A couple of minutes into the process: "Oh my God!"

I'm not sure which god Tracey was hailing, but it must have been the one that fixes severed NG tubes. Sure enough, Spencer walks out of the bathroom with two tubes when he walked in with one. Tracey appears behind him looking like she just stepped on Jim the Hamster. "We have to get a new one, Spencer. I'll call Eagle Ridge and see if they can put a new one in."

I'm going to preserve Spencer's sense of dignity and not explain what followed. Let's just say he was a little upset.

I have no medical training. If I see a bit of broken plumbing, it needs to be fixed. It wouldn't occur to me that you ought to rip all the plumbing out and start again. If it's copper, get a few connectors, solder in a new piece. That new-fangled fancy stuff, crimp in a new bit. If it's low-pressure plastic stuff and it only needs to be good for a few weeks and you don't have the parts?

Duct tape. Done. Two tubes were one again.

With duct tape, WD-40 and vice grips, you're pretty much ready for anything. I haven't had to use the vice grips or WD-40 on the boys yet, but they're ready when I need them.

Of Rabbits and Monsters

Yesterday morning arrived as a beautiful sunny day. We were all enjoying our coffee, cartoons, or what have you when the doorbell rang. Spencer went to get it and two of our neighbors were there. I was away in the office and heard only pieces of the conversation. There was much excitement and some discussion about a rabbit. I came to the door and suggested that we prepare the barbecue.

They had in their arms a cute little grey and white bunny. Apparently it was in our front garden being stalked by one of the neighborhood cats. They wanted to know if it was ours. It wasn't, of course. We barely have the skills to manage the one rodent we have.

Somehow or other, it was suggested that we should take this rabbit into our care. One of the finders had a terrier and the other was just about to go out of town. Oh lucky day, now we were rabbit owners. Why did they deprive the poor cat of a breakfast, interrupting the natural order? Ah well. Of life's great challenges, this one barely scratched the surface.

I darted into the office and retrieved my brand new trusty rodent trap. It was a small rabbit; I thought it would make a fine cage. The neighbors were clearly nervous at this point. I assured them that it would make a solid holding pen until I could get the barbecue ready. They left, somewhat reluctantly, more than a little unsure of my intentions.

Spencer disappeared into the kitchen with trap and bunny. In no time at all, he had lettuce out, a small dish of hamster food, and a fresh bowl of water. He was holding the bunny and had already determined that its name should be Cat Food. He sent me off to get the digital camera so that we could make little posters to put up around the neighborhood in hope of finding its real owners.

It was beautiful. The bunny was all about caring and kindness and love and hope.

Elsewhere in the kitchen, other things were brewing. Deep inside Spencer's body, the monster was back at work. His post MIBG scans on Friday showed new areas that were suspicious. His pelvis and spine and the original spots were all lighting up. As I've said, we don't like to practice amateur radiology, but this couldn't be good news.

This isn't beautiful. The monster is all about pain and suffering and uncertainty and fear.

So who wins this one? Caring and kindness and love and hope? Pain and suffering and uncertainty and fear? The rabbit is up against a tougher foe than the slow old tortoise.

It's a hell of a question. I, for one, don't want to know the answer. The only thing I know for sure is that tomorrow is going to be a beautiful day and I believe I'll skip work and go fishing with Spencer. On Wednesday, we'll go see the professional odds makers, and they no doubt will tell us that the monster has the edge. But that's two full days away. We'll give caring and kindness and love and hope a little head start before we go fighting monsters.

I think the rabbit deserves to win one.

Pumpkin Pie

Yesterday we began the traditional preparations for Thanksgiving. Well, pretty traditional. Just a couple of pumpkin pies. Actually seventeen pumpkin pies: four for the big family dinner, one for Spencer's friend Jared, and twelve mini pies for the nurses on the ward.

I began by gathering the required equipment and ingredients from home: some flour, a pot, mixing bowls, a few spices, brother Foster, pastry blender, and friend Jared. I packed them all in a bag and headed for the hospital.

Meanwhile, back at 3B, Tracey began the work of finding a kitchen. As it turns out, it's not an easy thing to do. She eventually found an oven somewhere on the second floor. The big problem was that Spencer couldn't leave his ward while the chemo was flowing so the playroom became our prep kitchen.

Tracey headed out to the supermarket to grab a few things I didn't bring. By the time you add up the milk, cream, pumpkin, mixing bowl, measuring cup, eggs, extra pie plates, measuring spoons, and spices, it was possible to get everything we needed for only $76 – just twice the price of what it would have cost to buy five pre-made pumpkin pies. It was a dead loss economically, but that wasn't really the point.

We gave the playroom table an alcohol bath and started the preparations. The secret, of course, is in the pastry. Real lard, very cold water, and a minimum of handling ensure the tenderest pastry. Needless to say, we rolled it to death. The filling had its final mixing in a washbasin and the first batch was ready for the oven. By this point, the chemo was finished and Spencer was free to leave the ward with his post-chemo hydration still hanging from the pole. Tracey took the boys downstairs while I started on the next batch up in the playroom.

In no time at all, the first batch was done and the second was ready for the oven. At this point the exercise became a little more complicated. Tracey had to run Jared home. I went down to the parking lot with them so I could have the parking pass to use with the car that uncle Johnny had dropped off so that we could deliver the pies when Spencer got a pass when his hydration finished. Then back up to Spencer's room, and he would lead me to the pies.

All was going well, right up to the point at which I headed back into the hospital with four minutes to spare and all the elevators were dead. So there I sat in the lobby with a boy all alone on the third floor and pumpkin pies in an oven at some undisclosed location on the second floor. It took me four different stairwells to find a path that took me to an open door on the third floor. I got to Spencer's room with no time to spare. Now, since he still had his IV pole, stairs weren't really an option. I was going to have to go solo. "Spencer, where are the pies?"

"Ah, I'm not really sure, Dad, but you know where we go to the lab? I think we turned the other way."

It only took me three stairwells to find one with a door open to the second floor. Now where? I had hoped that I could just go by smell, but it was tenuous. There was a faint odour of pumpkin radiating from the psychiatric ward. I tried there. There were no pies in Psychiatrics. Everything else on the second floor was locked up. Everything that was, except the Eating Disorders ward. Yes, it was here that I found an oven full of pumpkin pies, just ever so slightly overcooked. I'm going to have to think carefully this Thanksgiving about just what there is to be thankful for — there are just so many things.

Limping Along

There we were, indulging in the post-surgical euphoria. Spencer was recovering well. Most importantly, the bits of the beast were dead. There are those who have said that you have one clean shot at a cure. It's black and white. We were muddling around in shades of grey until that ever-so-brief pathology report told us that the world might be white after all. Life was good.

This disease makes us sensitive to our children. What does that cough mean? Why the persistent runny nose? How did you get that bruise? Everything has potential meaning. Our sensors seem to go up and down a bit depending on where we are in the cycle of treatments and how long it's been since the last scans and test results. Somehow, when he seems unbelievably healthy and it's been a few months since scans, an unexplained bruise brings a certain amount of terror. When you're doing well, there is so much more to lose.

After the surgery, he had every scan and test going and they'd had a look around on the inside and had a go at tissues under the microscope. Everything was clean. The monster was in full retreat. We could relax for a while. Our personal terror threat status had dropped to low for the first time in fifteen months.

Then it happened. Watching Spencer, you could see that his movements were a little guarded favoring his abdomen. It was nothing to worry about. He did, after all, have an eight inch incision that would take a while to heal. But then he seemed to have developed a limp. Personal terror threat status raised to yellow, or elevated.

"Spencer, why are you limping?"

"My heel hurts."

Ah, his heel hurts. The boy probably had a hard landing off his skateboard or bicycle or hang-glider or parachute or any of the myriad of other regular boy things he seems to have been doing since last week's hospital discharge. He probably jumped hard in the shallow end of a swimming pool by mistake. I've never heard of a case where the monster has come back with a vengeance and gone after the heel.

"So did you injure it in some way, Spencer?"

"No, it just hurts. I can't walk on it anymore." Those are danger words. Personal terror threat status raised to orange, or high. Over the next day or so, he became very reluctant to walk. When he did, he put no weight on his heel. Things seemed to be deteriorating rapidly.

Thank goodness for Tracey. She is a woman of action. She gathered up both the boys, Spencer with his sore heel, and Foster with his persistent cough, and took them off to the doctor. Interesting. A regular doctor. Our general practitioner. Someone unskilled in the oncological arts. If they had asked for an updated health history, I wouldn't see my family for three days.

When I got home from work that day, Tracey was furious. Deeply imbedded in the pad of Spencer's heel were three or four warts. The doctor had whipped out some magic wart killer stuff and applied it to his heel. When asked if it would hurt, he said no. Three hours later, Spencer was in tears with pain. There was no proper informed consent! No opportunity to explore other treatment options!

I laughed. That made Tracey angrier. Somehow, warts seemed like such an utterly normal everyday occurrence. Treat them all day long, any way you like, with or without proper consent. I can live with the consequences.

"And by the way, Foster probably has asthma and came home with a bunch of inhalers."

"Asthma? I don't really know anything about asthma. Is that worse than cancer?" Tracey's jaw dropped.

Personal terror threat status downgraded to green, or low. Husband status downgraded to doghouse.

Moving Up the Food Chain

I have just returned from Korea. Sometimes when travelling abroad, it is possible to have experiences that change your worldview and forever alter relationships with those you love. Such was my trip to Korea.

In all my travels to Asia, I think I have avoided drinking whiskey and singing karaoke. Not so this time. My selection was "Tie a Yellow Ribbon". It was badly sung, but the Koreans are such gracious people. They backfill with noisy cheers and tambourines so that nobody has to suffer. As traumatic as it was, there was nothing about singing karaoke that fundamentally altered my worldview.

No, it happened before that.

Mr. So and I arrived early for dinner. We were waiting for Mr. Kim, Mr. Lee, Ms. Park, and Mr. Su. We made idle chitchat. He explained to me that we would go to a special place for drinks later. He ordered up dinner and mentioned something about dark meat. I just nodded. I thought he said dark meat, but then again, Ks and Gs tend to be interchangeable in Korea, and Rs are soft.

Later, Mr. Kim arrived and sat down next to Mr. So. Now, I don't speak Korean, but I figure the conversation went something like this:

Mr So: "What took you guys so long?"

Mr. Kim: "Oh you know, the usual traffic. Have you already ordered dinner?"

Mr. So: "Yeah, I thought we'd go with dog tonight. I've ordered the sweet dog first and then the spicy dog for a little adventure."

Mr. Kim: "What are you, nuts? Westerners don't eat dog. We can't serve him dog."

Mr. So: "Oh, I just assumed given his skill with chopsticks and love of kimchi that he was fully integrated into Korean culinary habits. I told him we were going to have dog and he didn't mention that he had any problem with it."

Mr. Kim: "Now what do we do?"

Mr. So: "Let's not mention it. Maybe he won't know the difference."

When the spicy dog arrived, Mr. So said simply, "Ah, here is another kind of beef. A bit spicier than the first. I think you will enjoy it." Mr. So almost avoided one of those embarrassing international incidents.

But it was Mr. Su at the other end of the table whose curiosity became overwhelming. He asked in perfect English: "Is it common for people in Canada to eat dog?" Mr. Kim nearly choked on his kimchi.

Now I come home and see Scupper. I've always felt intellectually superior to him, but we shared a certain mutuality in our position at the top of the food chain. I can't help but wonder just how tasty he would be barbecued in little strips, served in lettuce leaves with a little chive, sliver of garlic and some tasty red chilli paste.

The Incident

I haven't been interacting with the world that much lately. We've kind of reached a point where we are socially withdrawn and avoid interaction with others due to the cloud of shame that hangs over our family. But alas, that is not my purpose in writing today.

I wanted to give an update on Spencer. He made it in just under the wire on the fenretinide study. There is a full series of scans and tests to be done prior to entry and it proved to be a logistical challenge to get it all done on time. The great news was his bone marrow was clean, one of the spots that was showing on the MIBG was gone, and the others had reduced in size from the two rounds of topless cyclone (topotecan / cyclophosphamide chemotherapy combination) that he had. The even greater news was that he is able to swallow the twenty-five or so monster fenretinide pills every day. This was no small feat as three months ago he couldn't swallow the smallest of pills. But as he explained to a seven-year-old girl in clinic who was admiring his prowess with a Septra tablet: "I used to have trouble swallowing pills. I tried practising with mini M&Ms. That didn't work so I took a three month break and now I have no problem." That was comforting, considering most of the other treatment options open to him involved stem cell rescue.

He has now started his second round of fenretinide and is doing great. No ill effects. He's in school. We've enjoyed great fun over the holidays: improving video game skills, cross-country skiing, generally fattening up, and growing hair. Life is good and whether warranted or not, we enjoy a cautious optimism as we move to another round of scans at the end of the month. It couldn't be better. Well, except of course for the cloud of shame.

It's the dog's fault. It started a few days before Christmas. The boys were at the annual Balding for Dollars sleepover beside the beluga whales in the aquarium. Tracey and I checked into a downtown hotel and enjoyed being adults. Scupper stayed with friends. While there, he managed to tear apart and eat his little rope Santa toy and eat the bits. He caused general mayhem. He's a dog. No shame in that.

No the shame came on Christmas Day. There were about twenty of us at my sister's gorgeous waterfront home for a turkey dinner. We were enjoying that post-meal euphoria. A few were lounging on the stairs that overlook the dining room. It was a perfect moment for that seasonal family photo. The rest of the group gathered round. The cameras were ready; the lighting was perfect. Even Scupper decided to join in the family photo.

It must have been something about the rich texture of the lovely white carpet in the dining room. When his feet touched it, Scupper felt compelled to drop his butt to the floor and drag it for several feet across the carpet leaving a three-foot deep brown skid mark. Apparently those stringy Santa toy bits were causing problems on the way out. It was unprecedented. We were speechless. The carpet was cleaned. Apologies were made. We hung our heads in shame and made our exit.

Eventually, in the fullness of time, we will get past The Incident and again be able to fully re-join society. Give us time. We are still tender.

No Redemption

Yesterday, I learned something from Scupper. To me, underwear is underwear. I don't have my favourite pair that I wear for special occasions. I don't have weekday underwear and bright colours for the weekend. I just have plain underwear and I like it all the same. Which is to say, I don't think about it all that much.

Yesterday, I learned that a woman, or best I not generalize on something like this, Tracey, has favourites among her underwear. There is a whole underwear spectrum to suit all occasions. Some is extraordinarily comfortable. Some is not. Why she doesn't just throw out the uncomfortable stuff and live a life of pure pleasure, I'm not sure.

At the top end of the favourite scale is her black bra. I won't claim to know what characteristics of the black bra make it her special favourite. It was only yesterday that I learned there was even a spectrum, a veritable scale of undergarment satisfaction.

Tracey was in the shower and Scupper came cruising through. He is more sophisticated than I am. He appreciates the characteristics of the black bra that led to its favoured position. He chose the black bra over the other articles of clothing lying in the bathroom, and it quickly became his favourite too. And like all his favoured things, he loved it with his teeth.

The black bra is no more.

Tracey says she would kill Scupper if he weren't so cute. Scupper is one bad haircut away from extermination. Yet somehow he charms and manages self-preservation.

I think the only thing worse than eating the black bra might be discussing Tracey's underwear with relative strangers over the Internet. I might be one email session away from extermination.

Car Repairs

The great thing about having a kid with cancer is it gives you a new perspective on life. There just isn't time to mess around with life's mundane details. I just received a bill for car repairs. It seemed high. It could be fair. I don't know and I don't care to waste my time finding out. Normally, the thing to do is pick up the phone, call the service manager, negotiate and straighten it out. I'd rather play Nintendo with my kids and not deal with the stress. This email to the service manager might be a little unfair, but occasionally, it feels good to share life's unfairness.

> *Hi Rod:*
>
> *It's been our pleasure to be customers of Westminster Volkswagen since moving to the area about a decade ago. We have a fine old Cabriolet that we love. It hasn't required much in the way of service, but the service it gets has been done largely in your shop.*
>
> *I would like to give you the opportunity to review the invoice referenced above. In my wildest imagination, I cannot think of how it might cost nine hundred sixty-two dollars and sixty-three cents to fix the windshield wipers.*
>
> *I buy the whole story about a leak in the fuse box and the need to replace a seal, which, by the way, you told my wife would be about five hundred dollars. I'm also fully cognizant that we had the door latch fixed. I'm generally a rational man.*

Unfortunately, your invoice doesn't detail the hours you spent. There is no way I can sit here and determine whether the price you are charging for the work you have done is reasonable.

Here is the really unfortunate part, Rod. My son has cancer. Every moment of my life is precious. I really don't have time to discuss details of obscure invoices and listen to the rationale that underlies them. I'm sure you have a good story. I also think if you review the invoice you may find an error that will reduce the price by two hundred dollars, bringing it down to the absurd edge of reasonable.

You can credit our MasterCard account by that amount or more and advise me by return email that you have done so. We will be pleased to continue our relationship with Westminster Volkswagen, albeit a bit more cautiously. I like having a place where we can drop the car and count on dependable service at a fair price. I'd like to get back there.

The alternative is to ignore this email and say this man is unreasonable and we would prefer not to do business with him anyway. I'm okay with whatever you choose. I just don't have the time to mess around.

Thanks So Much!

Steve

The very next day, they happened to be reviewing invoices and found an error on ours, which resulted in a credit of $229 to our MasterCard. Imagine that.

Life and Death and Warts

Monday was clinic day. The day we get the new prescription of fenretinide, review the official reports of all the scans, and ask all those serious questions. Oh yes, and of course we had to visit the dermatologist. The warts on Spencer's feet are back.

First the life and death stuff. We sat down with the dermatology resident. She had Spencer's chart, the full thick three inches of it. The other eighteen inches must be tucked away in record storage. We spend a long time going through history, describing all our wart related experiences. We get into wart theory. We have a deep understanding of the relationship between the immune system and warts. We go through the various treatment options. Though the modality of various treatments whether acid, or liquid nitrogen, or some kind of direct mechanical intervention, all differ, in the end they penetrate deeper into the skin and trigger the immune system to respond and attack the wart.

This is so much better than the nasty GP who splashed acid on his feet with not a thought about true informed consent. And this is just the resident. We're only preparing and laying the groundwork in anticipation of the staff dermatologist's arrival. We haven't yet begun to get serious about warts.

She arrives. It's not just clinical. This is a children's hospital. Spencer is an eight year old. He must be involved in the decision and has his own choices to make. How does he feel about having his warts cut away? Are they uncomfortable? Do they cause pain? Pros and cons all around. We've been treating with greasy Duoplant and it's hard to keep it contained to just the affected area. We had to stop because the adjacent skin was peeling away and becoming painful. Not treating the warts was presented as an option. My god, what were they thinking? Surely the warts will run rampant and my boy will become one massive wart. In the end, all the options are on the table and we decide to go with Soluver Plus. It sounds like a wonderful thing. Vincristine for the wart set with no loss of hair. Our boy will likely be saved and still enjoy a reasonable quality of life. No surgery. Very small chance of death due to a toxic reaction. Life is good. An hour and a half for warts.

Oh yes, then there was the meeting with the oncologist. There is no further progression. The CT scan is clear. The bone marrow is clear. The MIBG scan shows one of the spots is gone. The other is shrinking, maybe, but we can't find the last report because the chart has been cleaned out. Wasn't there a third spot? Whatever. We are on our way to lunch after five minutes for cancer.

It's bizarre and surreal. Our lives are full of high drama. A life and death turning point could come at any time, but then there are warts. It's a long string of events that is punctuated by moments of high expectation and terrifying fear, but there is no life and death turning point. Life and death are the same thing. They are served up together every day in small slices to chew on and savour or spit out in bitter rejection. One moment looks a lot like the one before and there's no telling exactly what the next will look like. We progress from one to the next with varying acceleration. It's pointless to look back. It's pointless to look too far ahead. It's pointless to sit in fear waiting for someone else to tell us how far we are from the destination.

So what's the point?

Enjoy the moment. They're all beautiful.

Seeing Clearly

Today I woke up and couldn't see out of one eye, and the image in the other was all blurry. A fine way to start the day. By the time I blasted my eyes in a hot shower, I could open them both and I was able to see again. In the mirror, I could make out the fine detail of all the blood vessels where the whites of my eyes used to be. It was perfect.

You're probably thinking this Steve guy needs to have his head rearranged—he keeps finding joy in all the crap that life throws at him. Why can't he just be miserable for once and scream, "Oh shit!"?

Normally, if my eyes were all infected and sore I would be miserable, but I am fortunate enough to have Spencer for a son. Last week when I took him in for a CT scan, one of his eyes was all red. I knew what it meant, and it had to be bad news. Surely disease had spread to his orbits and this was the first indication. What would follow? Black eyes? Almost certainly.

They humoured me at clinic and did not one, but two swabs. One viral and one bacterial. They even called the next day to advise that the bacterial swab tested positive. Do I trust that? Maybe. Spencer's eye seemed to clear up the next day with a few eye drops. It's fine now, but there was still that lingering doubt. But not anymore—I'm sure neuroblastoma is not contagious.

On the subject of scans, the news is mixed. The CT scan was clear. Bone marrow is clear. But the MIBG scan seems to have gone back to where it was last September. The same four spots, and of the same size. Radiology calls that progression. Oncology is not so sure. They say it's not necessarily bad news (though definitely not good news). If the spots were bigger or in different places, they would be sure, but they think maybe uptake of the MIBG on the last scan might have been blocked if it was occupied by residual treatment MIBG that was still present but not so radioactive. Sounds like a nice theory, but they were at a loss to explain it to me at a molecular level. For giggles, we did a bone scan on Friday and now await the results. It certainly looked frightening.

Now I'm no genius. I did however, once score 98% on a second year stats exam in nowhere near a state of sobriety. I know enough not to let hope triumph over probabilities, and the numbers suggest that it's a great time to enjoy a nice holiday on the beach in Mexico while we are all in good shape for snorkelling and have enough hair to block the harsh rays of sunshine. We leave on Sunday. We have plenty of time to do all this medical crap when we get back.

Oh shit!

Lunar Cycles

We returned from Mexico a week ago. The problem with vacations is that when you come back, reality is waiting for you.

I've been grieving. Our team is out of the playoffs.

They failed to put as many frozen turds in the other team's net as they put in ours, so now it's all over. There is scarcely any purpose in life without hockey. Not until next fall at least. We had a fantastic time in Mexico. We didn't tell the boys we were going until 5 o'clock on Easter morning when we woke them up to stuff them in a cab. We forgot to mention that we were two resorts down the beach from where Spencer's best friend Jared and his mom and dad, Jack and Donna were staying. They sort of discovered that the next day when we bumped into them as we walking down the road and their cab pulled over. We hung out together all week.

The beach was good. The boys spent eight hours a day in the water. If we weren't at the beach, we were at the pool. If we weren't at the pool, we were at a cenote. There was sailing and windsurfing and snorkelling and scuba diving and cliff jumping. We didn't all do those things. Some of them were dangerous, so I preferred not to jump off the cliffs.

I don't have to explain why my children now call me Rum Boy. The good news is they have stopped calling me Bock Bock Chicken Rum Boy. I shall never have to explain to you all what lunar cycles in a cenote are, but they do require a bit of rum and no swim trunks. I shall figure out how to delete the video footage and there will never be any evidence. Forget I mentioned it.

We managed to convince the sail boat guy that we were experienced in sailing catamarans in twenty knot winds with five foot swells and that he should let us take a boat out while all the others sat on the beach. We lost Jack's hat and Tracey went overboard when we turned the boat into a submarine after coming off the top of a wave. I know we recovered at least one of them. The other was lost forever.

When we came back, we wasted no time. It was clinic day. Our oncologist was a little concerned about the bruising under Spencer's arms. We had to explain that he had his arms extended on a few of the jumps and the bruising was from the impact with the water. This did not seem to relieve her. We thought it better not to mention that he went scuba diving. Boys will be boys, after all.

The plan going forward is very aggressive — we are taking the wait and see approach. Spencer started another round of fenretinide and we'll do another set of scans in three weeks to see what's what. From there, who knows? Perhaps something interesting that will involve stem cell rescue just so we can get that good clinical treatment feeling going again. Life has been way too easy for the last few months.

Unscheduled Terror

Today wasn't supposed to be scan day. Regular scan days have enough anxiety for my liking. Unscheduled scan days are downright terrifying.

It all started last week. We had spent the weekend on the sailboat in shorts and t-shirts. I left town to visit an aluminum smelter in a place where they had two inches of fresh snow. I had no idea that there were still areas of this country in the middle of winter. I didn't bring a jacket. Anyway, the whole trip was based on the assumption that Spencer's medical situation was stable and there would be no problem to pop out of town for a couple of days.

Assumptions are never really good things. When I left, Spencer had a sore neck. Probably pulled it playing road hockey, I thought. By the time I arrived in Montreal, it was bad enough that he was home from school. By the next day, he was in at Children's getting checked out. Probably just a pulled muscle, they say, but let's do a CT scan just to check if everything is all right. Assumptions are bad things.

I arrived back home in time for a very relaxing weekend. No stress at all. We had a wonderful Mother's Day. The boys and I planted a three-tiered basket with a random assortment of nursery plants and cooked a lunch for Tracey. We had dinner out followed by a walk in the woods. All very relaxing. No worries. Just a pain in the neck that seemed to be getting better.

Today he had the CT scan of the head and neck. They even promised us same day results. We never get same day results. This can't be a good thing.

But it was. Everything was perfectly normal.

So we can live the good life for a few more weeks until the next series of MIBG and bone scans. Those won't be perfectly normal, but in the meantime, Spencer has a birthday. He'll be nine.

Tracey had a brilliant idea for a party. She and Spencer decided on a workshop party. I loved the idea. Power tools mix well with eight and nine year olds. They delivered a dozen sandpaper invitations today.

I bought twelve little bottles of glue with eight-ounce hammers to go with them. Tonight Spencer and I started running rough lumber through the planer and table saw. We are going to kit up the parts for all the kids to build their own toolboxes. A toolbox filled with a hammer, nails, glue, and bits of wood makes a nice goody bag for a nine year old. It will be a testosterone-rich event. I thought I was clever, but I'm not.

One of Tracey's friends dropped by and said hello as we were exacerbating high frequency hearing loss and creating clouds of sawdust. When she found out what we were up to she broke into a smile. "Tracey's brilliant," said Leisa. "I could never figure out a way to have a birthday party and get Mike to do all the work!"

CONSOLIDATION

Con-sol-i-da-tion: 1) treatment given after induction therapy to mop up any cancer cells remaining in the body 2) that period of time where the child can't remember having hair and the parent can't remember having a mind 3) the stories of Spencer from age nine to age ten

No Humor; No Metaphor

Spencer has had a series of scans over the last few days and will have a bone marrow biopsy on Monday. It always takes several days before we get any results. We try to resist the urge to practice amateur radiology by looking at the low-resolution images over the tech's shoulder at the operator console. Nevertheless, we can't help ourselves and have refined our skills.

It appears that Spencer's disease progression is significant and very rapid. The technicians are not allowed to really say anything about what they see, but Tracey plies them with homemade cookies and maintains a close enough relationship that we are able to figure out what is going on in the limited conversations you can have in the room with Spencer and no authority to really say anything. During yesterday's bone scan, Tracey left to go to the oncology clinic to ask the doctors to be prepared to discuss the results and the plan going forward. "They are aware of the situation and we will talk on Monday." Doctor Lucy also gave Tracey a prescription for morphine tablets in case we need them over the weekend. I don't regard this as a very promising sign. I expect in Monday's meeting we will talk about how we deal with end-of-life planning for Spencer. I'm not sure about hopeful treatments.

Spencer has a pain in his hip, is having difficulty with stairs, and is stiff and sore. We haven't said anything to him yet until we know more, but he is a smart kid and probably knows that things aren't so good.

A Word from Steve

I may have used a term that I don't understand very well, but hey, that's okay. When we are where we are, I am allowed to screw up. I think some more clarification might be required.

I suggested that we might be discussing end-of-life planning for Spencer. I think I should be perfectly clear on what I meant by that because it probably has an entirely different meaning to somebody who's been farther down the road than we have.

Spencer is not a very sick boy who is trying desperately to cling to life in his final few days. We are not at the point where we are wrestling with what pain medications will make him most comfortable in those last moments. Last night he had a friend stay over. They've been running (and kind of limp hopping) around and playing hide and go seek. This morning they are playing soccer in the hallway and this afternoon we are going swimming at the local pool. Then Spencer is going bowling at a friend's birthday party. These are all things that he wants to do today, just like any other kid.

I do think that on Monday, we will find that there has very definitely been disease progression and that the Fenretinide is not working (or at least it's not working as hard as the neuroblastoma is). I also think that the oncologists may begin to discuss, for the first time, that we should also be thinking about treatment options that are directed at Spencer's quality of life and that we will have a number of important decisions to make that lead down a road that may forever rule out any chance of getting to NED (No

Evidence of Disease — remission). To me, that is a discussion about planning for end-of-life.

Does that mean we are just giving up? No. But it does mean that we have our ears open and we are going to want to think things through very carefully. When we have all the objective clinical data gathered on the scans and biopsy, you can be bloody sure that I'll be corresponding with one of the leading clinical neuroblastoma researchers in Los Angeles who happens to be amused by our story. We're dealing with a strong kid who still has buckets of stem cells and his brother is a perfect allogeneic match.

So what does all this mean?

Well, there is the rational Steve that understands very well the monster we are dealing with from a factual and probabilistic perspective. There is the emotional Steve who remains forever hopeful and optimistic. They don't always coexist in a harmonized way in my skull. Rational Steve would never buy a lottery ticket. Emotional Steve buys them all the time, but rational Steve never lets emotional Steve quit his job and run his credit cards to the limit in anticipation of the big win. What it means is that perhaps rational Steve and emotional Steve are going to open up a dialogue for the first time.

My God. Who is this other Steve who looks inside and can see them both and then write about them?

Congratulations on reading this far. It's going to take a little more bravery to continue, because the updates aren't always going to be full of cheerful Scupper stories any more. But hopefully they keep coming and we'll hear a word from rational Steve or emotional Steve or any of the other Steves that might rattle around from time to time.

No Big Deal

Spencer had his bone marrow biopsy this morning and we received news on the scans. There has been some significant progression of the disease. He has several areas in his pelvis lighting up, a spot in his left kidney, and some other areas up in his neck.

Obviously not good news, but it is certainly not as bad as it could have been. Nobody has given up or suggested that it is time to do so.

The immediate plan is to get him back on chemotherapy. He will be on chemo within the hour. The goal is to cool things down and get them back under control quickly. He'll be getting the topless cyclone again. This one isn't too evil in terms of the side effects and he can have it as an outpatient.

We expect he will receive a few rounds of this chemo and, depending on how it goes, we will likely be pursuing a more aggressive treatment. We don't know exactly what that will be yet, but we'll sort it out over the next little while.

It is never as bad as you think it might be, but never as good as you hope. Such is life.

Spencer is in good spirits. He didn't believe me when I told him his cancer was back and that Dr. Pritchard would be coming to talk to him about that and some more chemotherapy. He thought I was joking. Of course he was still kind of under the influence of ketamine at the time. When Dr. Pritchard did come, the reality set in. When he found out it would be topotecan and cyclophosphamide he was okay with that: “That’s no big deal.”

Dog Food

On Sunday, we had friends over for a lovely roast beef dinner. Last night, I wasn't sleeping well and came downstairs for a snack. I found some of that lovely left over roast beef. It was rather strangely packaged in one of those clear plastic containers that tomatoes come in. I thought that rather odd, since we have one of the largest Tupperware collections west of the Rockies. I grabbed a few bits right out of the box. It tasted okay, but the texture was kind of weird, as though it had been dragged through mashed potatoes. A chocolate cookie and glass of milk cleansed the pallet nicely.

Today I took Spencer to clinic for chemo. I wanted Tracey to have a break, go for a run, and spend some time with Foster. Dr. Lucy was impressed. Then she asked me a bunch of questions.

Dr. Lucy: "Did Spencer have a temperature last night?"

Steve: "No idea."

Dr. Lucy: "Did he take any more morphine yesterday?"

Steve: "No idea."

Dr. Lucy: "Did he have a dose of Ondansetron last night?"

Steve: "Umm."

She was impressed for only a brief period. Thankfully, Spencer was there to answer the questions. I guess my primary function in the clinic has been to play the games. I didn't realize that Tracey was doing all the work.

It was a quick dinner tonight and a rush to get Foster off to his T-ball game. Beef dip. Mmmm. As Tracey was putting the milk away, she pulled this strange package out of the fridge. It was that clear one with the roast beef in it. "If you're wondering what this is, it's food for the dog. Just the leftovers from people's plates on Sunday."

She could tell from the look on my face that it was too late. The boys thought it was hilarious.

I was tucking Spencer in to bed and Foster wandered in giggling hilariously. "Hey Dad. What's that thing on your butt? Oh look, it's a tail! Do you want some more dog food?"

They're still joking about it. I'm trying my best to pretend I'm angry at the teasing.

Father's Day

Every half dozen years or so, the planets align and Foster's birthday falls on Father's Day. At least I think it's every half dozen years or so; this is the first time it has ever happened. Spencer occasionally has his birthday on Mother's Day, or at least he did once.

It was one of those thoroughly exhausting weekends. We were out Friday night, and Saturday was a big T-ball tournament followed by a bowling birthday party, then off on the boat to Bowen Island. It was all go go go.

The rare moment of peace for me came this morning. I was up before everyone else. Everyone except Scupper, who had to pee. We went for a walk up to the coffee shop. I got a large cup of coffee to go. I think Scupper snuck in a few espresso shots. We went back to a large grassy area overlooking the cove in what I think might be the most beautiful spot in the world. I sat and enjoyed my coffee. Scupper played fetch with his tennis ball... relentlessly.

A beautiful young shepherdy-looking dog came and chased Scupper. She couldn't keep up with him. Her owner showed up shortly afterwards. He kept calling for her: "Come on Heidi, let's go get a coffee." I think all the men on Bowen Island like to hang with their dogs and drink coffee first thing in the morning. Heidi wouldn't come. She wanted to run with Scupper. I suggested that I would be there for a little while and if he wanted to go up and get a coffee, Heidi could hang with Scupper. He left a little bit reluctantly and went to get his coffee.

Well, about three throws later, Scupper had reached his thermal limit and disappeared over the rise and down to the beach. Heidi followed. They both came back several minutes later, absolutely soaking wet with seawater. Heidi's owner came back. "Sorry, I forgot to mention, Scupper is a rascal and a scoundrel. He took her for a swim."

"That's okay. I wanted her to learn how to swim anyway," he offered graciously. The rest of the crew eventually woke up and we all went out for breakfast before all the parents, brothers, sisters, and their families arrived on the ferry. We had a wonderful day picnicking in the shade, and hanging at the beach. I think Scupper retrieved the tennis ball about four hundred times before there were no fresh arms left. Spencer caught two fish off the dock. Foster saw a dead otter floating on its back. That was the highlight for him. Nothing like wildlife that doesn't try to run away from you. It gives you a chance for a good look.

Eventually we saw everyone off on the ferry and loaded up the boat for the return trip home. Scupper is a water dog and the obligations of his genes weigh heavily on him. He feels utterly compelled to patrol the boat and check on the well-being of the crew. He was on a continuous cycle—cabin to cockpit to foredeck to cockpit to cabin to cockpit to foredeck. He was driving everybody nuts. Finally, I tied a line to his collar and cleated him off in the cockpit. He stopped moving and dropped down with his head in Spencer's lap. And so we sailed home as the sun was setting.

In the car on the way back, the boys were fooling around. Somehow, and I'll never know exactly how, Foster ended up with a mouthful of Spencer's hair. It was all quite amusing for a few miles until he started coughing uncontrollably and puked up a hairball. I had to roll down the windows so we wouldn't be overcome with the smell.

That was our signal. Out came the clippers when we got home. Spencer and Foster are both near bald on the number one setting.

I opted for the shiny look of total baldness. Spencer will catch up to me soon enough. All the boys are bald of their own choosing.

As I tucked them into bed, we talked. We all feel that if Scupper could talk, he would tell us that he wants to be bald on the top of his head too. We'll get to him tomorrow. When I kissed Foster goodnight, he was wearing his new road hockey gloves.

Today was a fine Father's day.

Wingardium Leviosa

We live in Poco, a suburb where they celebrate Canada Day with a big fireworks display two blocks from our house in Castle Park.

We made a few scouting missions over the course of the day. The RCMP maintain quite a presence to make sure that law and order are upheld. I must say that when they see an electric go-kart with a big Canadian flag, they obviously struggle with what is being violated: law or order. As long as Spencer kept driving, at low speed and without knocking down pedestrians, they seemed happy to be left pondering rather than having to deal with it. I'm quite sure there would be at least a half day of questions and paperwork to arrest a nine-year-old boy for driving an unregistered vehicle on the sidewalk without a driver's license. For my part, I will maintain that it is not a motor vehicle, but an electric wheelchair. In any case, we managed to get through the day without even being questioned. No tickets or arrests.

The big event was, well, exactly what you would expect from a suburban fireworks display. Definitely better than you could achieve in your backyard, but not exactly the Symphony of Fire. When the boys arrived home, they had obviously not reached their saturation point for seeing glowing lights fly through the air.

Tracey bought them the little eighteen-inch glowing tubes of chemical soup. They now come packaged in an aluminum tube so they aren't accidentally activated in shipping and handling. It started as a Harry Potterish thing. Stuff the glow stick into the tube, brandish it in a large arc while reciting "Wingardium Leviosa", and light emerges from the wand. Do it a little quicker and it shoots out of the wand across the back yard. It was fun, but somewhat uncontrolled. They tended to land on the roof, fly over the fence, or knock over my drink. A better solution had to be found.

Luckily, I just happened to have a fifty-foot air hose for the compressor that reaches nicely out to the patio. When mated to the aluminum tube, it makes an excellent glow stick cannon. We were able to easily achieve sixty-foot altitude. Bright streaks of vertical fluorescent fire would shoot into the air and then come tumbling back to earth. It was at least four times as much fun as the fireworks display at the park. After several shots, we noticed quite an interesting phenomena. The glow sticks would shoot up and then come back down, then, strangely, they started travelling in rapid bouncing horizontal motion about two feet off the ground. It was most unusual.

Anyway, if you want to try this at home, you will need:

- Glow sticks and tubes
- Air compressor
- Rubber tipped blow nozzle
- Portuguese Water Dog (black is best)

Pediatric Weaponry

We've completed an upgrade on Spencer's go-kart. I just sent an email to our friend Will, who is an RCMP officer. It read as follows: "Will: We installed the dog ball fetch assist device on Spencer's electric wheel chair. It turns out that it is tremendous saving for Spencer's energy, what with his chemotherapy and all. It would normally take him about five throws to get it to go the 150 m distance. Now he can do it by pressing just one little button. Medical assist devices have advanced so much with modern technology."

It's probably best not to tell law enforcement officials that the all-terrain electric assault vehicle that Spencer's uncles designed and built has now been outfitted with artillery. I was inspired by the shooting glow sticks and couldn't help myself.

Now Spencer has three new switches: "Compressor", "Arm Weapons", and "Fire." It makes an awesome noise and shoots a tennis ball an unbelievable distance. Scupper just hears a "wumph!" and has no concept that his beloved tennis ball is just re-entering the atmosphere after a brief low-Earth orbit. This is going to take a bit of training. We'll have to work on lower pressure shots so that he can see the tennis ball and associate the cannon firing—pardon me, "fetch device activation"—with his tennis ball.

It also does a fair job with water balloons. It's possible to load a half dozen small ones in the barrel and fire it across the street, over the neighbour's house, and soak the neighbour in his back yard. I think it's possible to have more fun, but I would probably have to do something illegal. Oh, never mind.

Oh yeah, and there is that whole medical thing. Spencer finished his second round of topless cyclone on Friday. We're just hanging out waiting for his counts to drop. He's in great shape and went for an hour and a half hike today to swim under a waterfall. He certainly has no disease symptoms and tolerates the chemo well. I hope it's doing some good. We'll talk to the oncologist this week about more aggressive therapy and do another set of scans in few weeks to see where his disease is. In the meantime, we play hard.

Preparing for the Inevitable

Somehow, I thought if I was strong and confident, we could keep things in control. Little by little, it starts to slip away. It doesn't take a genius. I can see it coming. You hear about it, but you believe it won't happen to you. Then you're just down to hope. After a while, that's not enough so you try to believe in miracles.

I can see now that this one is not going to go my way.

We started out with the best of intentions. We were going to contain it. We were going to be different than the others.

It doesn't happen all at once, of course. It's little bits here and there. Gradually the tide turns, and there's nothing you can do to stop it from coming in short of reversing the moon.

Our dog was not going to be allowed outside the family room. He was going to make his life there on the washable cork floors and out in the backyard. No kitchen. No living room. No dining room. No bedroom. And definitely no drinking out of the toilet. At night, he would sleep in his crate.

We put up one of those baby gates to keep him contained. Eventually, we all just got tired of stepping over it every time we went to the kitchen or upstairs. Oh, let the dog in the kitchen, but not at mealtimes! And definitely not in the living room on the carpet.

Guess who started hanging out in the kitchen during mealtimes?

Yes. Scupper. I growl at him and he goes away. So while we eat, he lays down on the living room carpet. This takes way too much energy.

Sleeping in the crate? Not so much any more.

We draw the line. All right, he can go where he likes downstairs as long as he doesn't hang out at the dinner table and he doesn't go upstairs.

So every night when we're all upstairs reading stories, I can hear the dog creeping up the stairs. I storm out of the room and yell things at him. I don't even bother with English any more. Anything that sounds tribal, frightening, and dominant alpha-male like seems to do the job. He runs back downstairs.

But it's wearing off. Now he only goes a couple of steps down and sits and waits stubbornly until I wave my arms and tell him to go all the way down in my best Klingon dialect.

Tonight, as I came out of Foster's room, I saw him sitting there on the top step. As far as he is concerned, if he hasn't taken that last step, he is still downstairs because he is not all the way up. It's like he went to some damn canine law school.

I know what he's doing. I know where this is going. It's only a matter of time.

It could happen any time. It could happen tonight. I'll probably find him curled up on my side of the bed, and when I start screaming at him in some Java dialect, he'll probably growl at me, and Tracey will wake up. There will be a suggestion that for the peace of the household, it might be better if I just slept downstairs.

In the darkness of night, it will be a little cool, so I'll grab the dog blanket and pull it over me to take the chill off.

I'm prepared for the inevitable.

A Boy in Japan

Today was bone scan day. I always find it to be a terrifically frightening experience, so I don't really look at the operator's console, but Tracey did. She bribed the technicians with muffins and bravely probed for results while Spencer and I were out of the room. We'll see what the official word is whenever they have it.

As for last week's CT scan, we did get official word, which was as follows: "The CT scan was better! His left kidney is now completely normal and there is some improvement in some of the bone lesions. The original mass on the right looks the same. I do not have the written report yet but we went over the scan carefully in XR rounds. So I think that is good news and we will continue with the cyclo/topo for now."

Which is very encouraging. We were sure the chemo was working, and I think most of the coastal villagers subject to his pillaging over the weekend would likely agree. We do know though, that the chemo is not going to work forever and give him a cure. It will slowly have an increasing impact on his bone marrow and they will have to go with lower doses and longer intervals between rounds. At some point, the cancer will decide to have a party again.

Which brings us to the subject of the discussion we had last week. Later on in the fall, Spencer will likely have another aggressive treatment. The one currently favoured by his oncology team is what they call an allogeneic transplant. What this means is that they will hit Spencer hard with a large dose of chemotherapy of one kind or another and perhaps total body radiation. This will completely wipe out his bone marrow. He will then be rescued with Foster's bone marrow. Along the way, he will develop some measure of "graft versus host" disease, which sounds nasty and dangerous, which of course it is, but it is hoped that the new bone marrow will also go after the cancer. There will be some kind of huge fight going on inside Spencer with no guaranteed winner, though we know who we will be cheering for.

It's all rather experimental and far from proven. The good news is that there is a boy in Japan who did the same thing and is alive and well and cancer free. So that's what we are down to: one boy in Japan.

This is not the only option for treatment and the oncology team will support us if we want to do something different. I can't say the other options are any more promising, and mostly they would happen far from home. Tough decisions. I had hoped four days of sailing would give us clear answers on what to do. I think the only conclusion we reached is that it would be nice to go sailing again.

Living Soundly in Desolation

There was no Scupper. He wasn't allowed on the charter boat, and there were no shortage of volunteers to look after him at home, even with full disclosure.

There were eagles and otters and giant red jellyfish. There were dolphins and seals. Fresh prawns for dinner. There was the barbecue that tried to commit suicide in the middle of Waddington Channel, and a cougar sighting ashore that left us a little reluctant to let our children wander the beach looking like small prey animals.

There was water so warm that we would have to go to Mexico to find anything like it on this coast. We went swimming every day, and some nights too, with glow sticks attached to the boys' swim trunks, and no compressor to shoot them in the air.

We hiked to beautiful freshwater lakes through carpets of thick green moss that made you want to lie down and have a nap. With very few bugs.

There were waterfalls pouring down breathtaking mountains that taste like no other after a long hike up.

We saw the harmless looking little channel that connects Squirrel Cove to a big lagoon, which on a rising tide sucked us in our dingy and our friends in theirs into a lagoon only to work our way back along a barnacle encrusted shore with only three pairs of shoes between seven of us. Thank god for warm water, a beautiful sunset, and two hundred feet of rope.

Later we had popcorn on the foredeck, with ice cold beer, under unbelievable starry skies. The kids were asleep in their bunks as we watched and cheered the stragglers who declined our rescue offer emerge from the lagoon at slack tide while meteors fell.

There was a long sandy beach with shells and driftwood — my new coffee table in kit form, waiting to be assembled with no instructions other than the memories.

Chocolate with friends. Milk and dark and dark with almonds, and ice cream from a miraculous invention that I've never experienced on a boat — a freezer.

We fished in a small dingy with the threat of rain and two hundred fifty pound halibut, neither of which materialized. But there were Cheetos and beer and friendship.

I think perhaps George Vancouver was having an off day when he named it Desolation Sound.

When we came home, we had a dog so happy, I thought he might vibrate out of his woolly alpaca coat.

The boys were so happy to see their dog that, just this once, was allowed to sleep upstairs.

An Update from Scupper

The big one kept me locked out of the room all night. I'm trying to interface my dog dish on the wireless network, but I can't seem to get it to communicate properly, so I can only write when he is snoozing on the couch watching the Olympics.

Anyway, things are shockingly normal around here. Spencer is home all the time and playing with his friends and doing kid stuff. Recently, I've been teaching them synchronized diving. We all line up on the edge of the boat and Spencer says, "Ready, Scupper?" at which point I jump overboard. Then Spencer counts "1,2,3, go" and he and Foster jump in behind me. The boys just need to work on jumping in a little sooner and not waste all that time counting. When they get better at it, I must say I like our medal chances. The big guy just seems to laugh and take pictures through all of this. He's not much of a coach.

That Foster kid is really growing up fast. He's six now and about to start first grade. He's amazingly tough. He has legs like a tree trunk and is strong from all the beatings that Spencer and his friends give him. He always seems to be laughing and smiling and there is not much in this world that bothers him. He just needs to follow my instructions a little more closely.

The Spencer kid is amazing. He is a sweet boy full of energy and smart like a whip. I think he has missed about half of his formal education, but he is still near the top of his class even though all his instruction is in French and we only speak Dog and English here at home. He starts grade four in a couple of weeks. Even though he doesn't have any hair, the other kids all like him and he has really good friends. His buddy Jared even goes to the clinic with him sometimes while he has chemo, just because he likes hanging out with Spencer. I go to the clinic sometimes too, but I have to stay out on the patio because they won't let me go inside.

Tracey is amazing. She understands me like none of the others. She is the boss of everything and makes the whole family run. Don't tell the big guy. She has enough love for everybody and a firm hand to keep us all going in the right direction. Without her, all the other ones would be in big trouble. She even does all the medical stuff and tells all of Spencer's doctors what to do.

I worry about Spencer. He is a normal kid and everything. I don't think anybody ever told him that when you are sick, you're different from everybody else, so he never figured it out and just carries on being a kid. But he still has that cancer thing happening. He's had topo/cyclo all summer long. Spencer calls this "easy chemo". It's making his tumor bits shrink and that is good, but the big ones are mumbling about kicking everything up a notch. They're just waiting for Spencer to start in the first week of school and meet his new teacher and establish a place to be and then I think they are going to start hitting him hard with bigger treatments. I think they want this cancer thing to go away. I hope everything works out okay.

As for the big guy, he's a pain in the arse. He still does his "dominant alpha male" thing and tries to tell me what to do. He thinks he's smarter and stronger than me. I humor him, but practice passive aggression. Usually I just find something good to chew on and drive him a little crazy. I have fun at bedtime. They try to shut me in the family room, but when I hear them getting ready to go to bed, I run into the living room and hide under the coffee table and pretend I don't understand what they want. This drives the big guy nuts. It's going to take a while, but eventually I will wear him down and I'll be allowed to sleep upstairs with my boys, as it should be.

Anyway, I keep working on the training. Eventually I'll have them all whipped into shape and everything here will be exactly as I want it. I just need to be patient and persistent.

Imponderable Questions

The boys started school today. Okay, so it was only a half hour. Foster has moved on to Grade 1; Spencer is in Grade 4. They reported to their old classrooms and their presence was duly noted. Tomorrow is the real deal. New teachers, a full day with a bag lunch. Tracey won't know what to do with herself.

We were camping on the weekend. There were friends there who had the new Gameboys with the flip-up screen. I don't remember having a Gameboy when I went camping as a kid. I think we may have had sticks, and if we were lucky, some string. Spencer decided he had to have one. I was thinking perhaps for Christmas. Spencer was thinking today.

We did the math last night. The boys had rolled up all the loose change in the house. They got to keep 25% between them. It was a good math lesson. Spencer can now figure out what 12.5% of anything is. With the contents of his wallet and the rolling fee, he figured he had enough money. I figured he was maybe $30 short. He wanted his 12.5% in bills right away. I told him no problem; he just has to take all the coin rolls to the bank. He persuaded Tracey to drive him. Can he buy the Gameboy now?

He would gladly mortgage his brother for immediate gratification. As far as he can tell, money has no intrinsic value. It's only good if it flows through his hands as though pressurized. I told him he would have to wait until he saved enough. I could hold out for months.

I didn't count on Spencer. He went to his favourite wheeler-dealer, Pokémon card selling, used CD, video swap-and-shop store across from the bank. He traded in his perfectly good Gameboy for an ultra-cool one with a backlit flip screen and didn't have to con another dollar out of his mom or pawn his brother. He seems to have no problem living life in the moment.

Foster lives at the other extreme. He has hundreds of dollars saved up. He could have wandered into the same store and bought three new Gameboys, but he won't part with a dollar. He has ambitions to be wealthy. We ride by expensive homes, and he says he is going to buy one for us one day. For some reason, I don't doubt it for a minute. We'll have to do a different math lesson with him: Interest calculations.

One boy lives for the moment, the other one has a long-term plan. Why is that? I don't want to know, but have no inclination to correct either one.

As we were getting ready for bed tonight, Foster was thinking about school and the long-term plan. "When I'm in Grade 6, will Spencer be in Grade 10?"

Wouldn't that be nice? I answered, "No Foster, he'll be in Grade 9."

"So will we be able to walk home from school together?" he asked.

"Won't you be in different schools?" I wondered.

"No, we'll both be in middle school," he assured me.

"Then you can walk home together." Wouldn't that be nice, Foster? I sure hope so.

Prepping for the Game

Both boys had their first soccer game of the year. Spencer played his full game. The coach subbed him off regularly in the first half, but by the second half, he was waving the coach off to sub somebody else out instead while he did double shifts. I guess his hemoglobin is where it should be. I think they won the game something like six or seven to nothing. Today he went to school.

When things are going well, that must mean it is time to pick on him again. Tracey and I met with his oncologist today. Tomorrow he gets admitted to the hospital. This time it will be cisplatin and VP-16. These are two of his least favourite chemos. Last time he had them, he lost ten pounds and about 40% of his high frequency hearing. The good news now is that he doesn't have as much hearing to lose and ten pounds doesn't mean 20% of his body weight any more. He's really in great shape.

The plan is to do this for two consecutive rounds and then follow it up with a full set of scans in late October, followed by transplant sometime in early November. It's hard to say what the timing will be exactly.

All of this will require an upgrade to his plumbing. I just spoke with the surgeon's office. They had a cancellation on Wednesday so he will have surgery late that afternoon to put in a double CVC (central venous catheter) as a replacement for his single VAD (venous access device). That means he gets a couple of tubes connected to his bloodstream that hang out of his chest. We will be back in the business of dressing changes and heparin injections. No more swimming, and he probably will be a little reluctant to take a soccer ball in the chest.

Anyway, the chemo will run until Friday afternoon. His doctor is in no hurry to kick him out until Monday, but we'll see how it goes. He might escape for a few hours on Sunday for soccer photos.

The prime objective is to avoid the barf fest. Tonight we picked up a prescription of Nabilone. This is synthetic marijuana in tablet form. He gets some tonight and some tomorrow. He will be at school for the first hour. It should be interesting as he sits at his desk going, "Oh wow man..." as he munches on Doritos. They gave him ten pills and he'll only use two. I guess the rest are for me.

Clinical Trials

Today, as we enjoyed what seems like the umpteenth day of hospitalization, we were advised that Spencer would need a nasal gastric tube tomorrow if he wasn't able to eat and drink in reasonable quantities to arrest the weight loss that started with his last round of chemo. But they were very fair about it. He was offered a little bit of Nabilone to stimulate his appetite.

He took it about a half hour before Uncle Johnny left. We had good fun playing in the hallway with the small solar power car kit that Spencer hot-wired with batteries so he can run it indoors.

All was going well until the Nabilone kicked in. Spencer developed a profound interest in a wheelchair that was lying in the hallway. He sat in the chair and worked the brake levers back and forth. Back and forth. Back and forth. He was driving a tank. We said goodbye to Uncle Johnny as Spencer sat in his tank.

The imaginary tank was quite captivating for a time, but eventually he craved the motion. "You push my IV pole, Dad. I'm going to drive this thing." During his struggles, he managed to run over one of his IV lines. Three others got tangled in his wheels. I had to put a stop to the whole exercise.

We went back to the room and decided to watch a DVD. His selection was *Looney Tunes: Stranger Than Fiction*. Usually, he's quite sophisticated in his tastes, but he began giggling uncontrollably watching Daffy Duck and the Tasmanian Devil. The munchies kicked in and he desperately wanted me to get him something to eat, but he couldn't tell me what he wanted as he was giggling so hard. In the end, he sent me for cookies.

I know as a parent, I should find such behaviour mildly disturbing. In truth, I found it all rather funny. It would be enough to make me question whether I am a good parent or not, except last weekend I undertook actions on behalf of my child that leave me assured that I am a good Dad.

You see, last time I mentioned Nabilone, a kind soul managed to source for us a large box of what can best be described as Nabilone cookies. Except they are herb-based rather than refined chemicals. They were represented as a better alternative to the capsules as they are more effective at stimulating appetite and reducing nausea while being easier to regulate dosage.

I am pretty sure the cookies didn't come from a pharmacy. There was no instruction label. I was told that about a half cookie was purported to be the right dose for a seventy-year-old woman roughly twice Spencer's size. I took them home and put them in the freezer as instructed.

I gave them no further thought until Friday night. I put Foster to bed and was quietly watching TV when my thoughts turned to Spencer. There he was, lying in a hospital, hardly eating much of anything and wasting away. Sitting in my freezer was something that might be able to help him.

But I had a major problem. Without the instructions from the pharmacy, how would I know what dose to give him? I could not subject my child to this kind of risk.

I did what any good parent would. I undertook a phase one clinical trial right in the comfort of my own living room. First, I started with the study design. Normally in a phase one trial, we want to slowly increase the dose and observe toxicity. Now, it wasn't like we had a clinic full of test subjects. After all, there was only me. Well, and Scupper of course.

But if I killed the dog, they would kill me, so I had to limit eligibility for the trial to a single subject. I figured it this way: I'm maybe three times Spencer's size. If somebody twice Spencer's size took a half cookie, then the correct dose ought to be about three quarters of a cookie for me, which would scale down to a quarter of a cookie for Spencer.

In the interest of accelerating the trial and maximizing the benefit, I set my dose at two cookies.

The clinical summary? Oh wow, man. To say I've never experienced anything quite like it would of course be a lie.

I've never experienced anything quite like it. At first, I was quite functional. I did a bit of email. It started to seem a little strange after a while. I decided to call my sister to work out a problem with logistics for taking the dog and Foster on the ferry to visit with Auntie V. She reduced an intractable complicated challenge to a simple solution in no time. Pure magic. I decided to watch a little TV. I have no idea what I watched or how long I watched it, but it was really good.

After ten minutes or two hours, I'm not entirely sure, I started to get very hungry. Tracey was probably wondering what happened to all those cookies she baked. They're gone. All I can say is, thank goodness I didn't get my cookies confused, or there would have been a nasty spiral that would have eliminated the entire contents of the refrigerator.

Eventually, I got very tired and went to bed. When I woke up in the morning, I would like to say that I was alert and refreshed. This would be another lie. There appears to be a big a difference between inhaling and ingesting. This of course based on what they tell me; I don't have any first-hand experience. When you ingest, it seems to stick with you for a long time. I did manage to get the coffee made eventually. Breakfast was superb. I had several bowls of Cinnamon Toast Crunch with Foster.

Obviously, the clinical trial was an outright failure. In my ambition to achieve quick results, I ramped through dose escalation much too quickly and executed with a poorly designed protocol. Now I'm going to have to start the whole trial over again.

We do what we have to for the well-being of our children. If it turns out that there are no cookies left for Spencer, so be it. I can't expose him to unnecessary risk.

Date Night

Last night was date night. The height of romance. It had all the attributes of a perfect evening: a little excitement, undressing, a small bed with fresh sheets. But I shouldn't go into all the details.

It wasn't the usual sort of date night. After all, Spencer was only out on day parole. He had to go back to the hospital.

That didn't stop me from including all the romantic touches. At Costco, I picked up a bunch of flowers to go with the jug of milk and the tomatoes. Not to mention a new shirt. I was looking spiffy. Tracey reminded me that we weren't supposed to have cut flowers in the house when Spencer's counts were so low. I think she threw them out.

We had our dinner together at home for the first time in a long time. We even had friends over. In our keenness to make sure that we didn't miss our planned movie, we left poor Tonya loading the dishwasher and folding laundry as we rushed out the door with the boys. Fine hosts we are.

Our first stop was Children's Hospital. We had arranged for Auntie Vicki to watch the boys while we went out and enjoyed the show. We got everyone settled in and we were on our way. Alone at last. All was well.

There was a small problem. As we made our way over the speed bumps and out of the hospital parking lot, the pain in my chest, which had been bothering me off and on all day, became quite a lot worse. I woke up in great discomfort on the hospital cot that morning. The pain seemed centered on my heart and radiated up into my neck and shoulder on the left side. I reached the conclusion that there was no way I could sit through a movie. I was in agony.

Rather than simply dying and leaving Tracey in a terrible pickle, I suggested that we turn right and head for Vancouver General Hospital rather than turning left and going to the movie theatre. She was agreeable. Nothing like a little adventure on date night.

The service at the hospital was really quite good. When you wander in as a nearly forty-ish male clutching your chest, they don't leave you waiting all that long. Spencer and I have a long running joke that nurses are easy to identify because they can't help but slap a blood pressure cuff on you and take your temperature. They didn't disappoint, and it wasn't long before they started diving into my health history.

"Have you experienced this pain before?" — No.

"Any problems with your heart?" — No.

"Cholesterol okay?" — No idea.

"High blood pressure?" — Don't think so.

"Any history of heart problems in the family?" — Yes, father.

"Been under any stress lately?" — Not that I can think of.

Tracey stopped them there. "We do have a child on the oncology ward at Children's." I conceded that one. Some minor stress.

"Are you on any medications?" — No.

"Any recreational drug use?" — Uh, um, no (Scupper wasn't there to betray me).

It wasn't long until they had little foil pads firmly stuck on all the hairy bits of my body and wired up to their machine. I didn't cry when they took blood. Spencer would have been proud.

Tracey was disappointingly calm. It seems nothing can bother her anymore. We sat on a little stretcher in a waiting area watching people. An emergency room on a Saturday night is quite an interesting place. Ambulance drivers would come in and drop off their charges. We decided to make the best of our date and enjoy the people watching. There were a few annoying people who came in. One guy was claiming that his father had just had heart surgery and wasn't feeling well. An obvious attempt to jump ahead of us in the queue. Oh well. One of the ambulance drivers had an amazing toupee—quite breath-taking.

Eventually the maître d' admitted us to the general emergency room. No more cocktails in the lounge. He had a little booth for us far away from the kitchen and he introduced us to our waiter, Tony. Tony was a great guy. You could tell he was used to working in the high priced places. Not too intrusive and in your face, but attentive nonetheless. He advised that our blood work would be up shortly and that he had booked a chest X-ray for me. No need to look at the menu. Then he went about sticking a new set of electrodes on me, trying to avoid the hairy bits. "Oxygen saturation is 97%, would monsieur care to try a little bit from the tube and see if we can get it up to 100%?" Very thoughtful. And of course, blood pressure and temperature.

Tony had that quiet way about him. He pointed out the EKG looked fine, just a little something unusual here. "You see how it goes bump bump and then a little pause and then a bump then a pause and a bump bump?" Nothing to worry about though.

Now since you don't generally expect emergency room personnel to say something like, "Holy crap, this looks bad, can you hang on for a minute while I get the crash cart?" his words were quietly terrifying. I guess this is how they tell you you're having a heart attack. Kind of ease you into it gently so they don't make a bad situation worse.

The X-ray guy came around to take me for my chest X-ray. He asked me many questions that really seemed directed at making sure I didn't keel over while I was under his care. I found this whole experience absolutely terrifying. The last time anybody in my family had a chest X-ray, we got to meet pediatric oncologists for the first time. I wondered if I would still have any good days left and how Tracey would be able to manage after they found the huge mass in my chest that was causing all this pain. Eventually, my X-ray tech rolled me back and reunited me with my sweetheart.

I thought the date was going rather well at this stage. Tracey seemed to be enjoying herself. It was kind of nice to be away from the kids and Children's Hospital and just have some quality time together.

Eventually, the doctor came around. She asked me many questions trying to get me to describe the pain I was in. "Uh, um, it hurts, like here and here. Sort of like a back spasm that won't go away." Of course, by this time, the pain pretty much did seem to be going away. It's just like when you go to the mechanic and try to get your car to make the same noise again.

"Are you aware that you have a sinus arrhythmia?" Hmmm, no. Okay, so this is how they tell you you're having a heart attack, but she seemed so nonchalant about it. These people are real pros. This would be very low key and matter of fact. I don't know why they won't just tell me. It's not like we're not equipped to deal with bad news. They have no idea that we are professionals.

Anyway, it was one of those surreal moments. Tracey kept persistently questioning to find out how bad this sinus arrhythmia really was. To me it sounded like I was blowing my nose out of key, but apparently it's nothing to be concerned about.

My blood was normal. The enzymes would have shown up by now if I had a heart attack. I had no tachycardia, which is apparently the really bad news even though it sounds less scary than a sinus arrhythmia. My pain symptoms were more consistent with something muscular than heart related. It looked like maybe I was home free. She just had to check the chest X-ray before we could go.

There was only a few minute delay while we waited to find out about the huge mass in my chest. Then to my relief, the doctor came back and announced the X-ray was perfectly normal. We were free to go. We thanked them for their excellent service.

Elapsed time? About two hours. Pretty much the same as a movie. But somehow it seemed much more engaging than a regular film. I was keen to start planning our next date, though Tracey thinks it was all done just so I could write about it. Somehow, when I was lying in pain at 3:00 this morning, I didn't feel like writing.

When we got back to Children's, the nurses were all interested to know how our movie was. We just smiled. They laughed as though they knew we had just come back from a hotel that charges by the hour.

Shoe Size

I was sick on Friday. I watched everything there is to watch on TV.

I used to love home improvement shows, but now they are all reality based, which means of course that they are unreal. The victims are removed from their houses while forty people do a shoddy job renovating their place in three days. I can't bear to watch them anymore. Whatever happened to Norm? Now the only good shows on television are the ones where they fabricate hot rods and motorcycles. I have to learn to weld.

The boys returned home from school on Friday afternoon. Since there was a gap in decent programming, no *American Chopper* or *American Hot Rod*, we watched a documentary on shoes on the Discovery Channel. It was quite excellent really. It covered everything from 5000-year-old shoes to modern Nikes. Biomechanics of ballet and soldiering. Testing from grip to electrical shock at 15,000 volts. Very informative.

I'm not entirely sure why, but the producers of the show felt compelled to bring up the relationship between shoe size and penis size. It was one of those awkward moments. You think you're watching family programming and then they take you over the hairy edge. What to do? If you change the channel, penis size becomes one of those forbidden taboo subjects of great interest. So we just continued watching.

The topic was well-researched. In general, there is some loose relationship between the sizes of the body's appendages, but there is no strong correlation between shoe size and penis size. The strongest correlation they have found is with the span between tip of index finger and thumb when the hand is fully extended.

Eventually it passed and they went on to talking about the finer points of leather. We were safely through it. No questions from the boys. They probably weren't even paying attention. I wasn't going to have to explain anything. That was good.

Later on, Tracey decided to take Spencer and Foster out to a movie with their friend Michael. They picked up Michael and were driving to the theatre. In the back of the car, the boys were all very busy comparing the span of their hands from tip of index finger to tip of thumb.

They were paying attention.

Most Valuable Player

The coach called last week. He had kind inquiries about my cardiac status, but that wasn't the real purpose of his call. He had managed to fill in that unnecessary break in the soccer schedule over the Thanksgiving weekend. He had found a tournament for the team to play in. There would be four soccer games: two on Saturday and two on Sunday. Would Spencer be up for it?

I suggested that we would at least try to attend a few of the games. I didn't know if Spencer would be ready to play. After all, he had spent most of the last month on his butt in the hospital and has a new set of plumbing hanging out of his chest. The coach suggested we dress him anyway and if he wanted to play, he would play him.

I asked Spencer if he wanted to play in a soccer tournament on the weekend. He didn't pause to think about it or wonder how he would do. His immediate response was "Sure!" It's not good to underestimate Spencer. He has a habit of surprising.

Saturday morning rolled around. I had picked up some kind of bug and spent the night alternating between shivering uncontrollably and soaking the sheets in sweat and didn't make it out of the bed for the first game. I don't quite have the character of my son. Tracey took the three boys to the game. Apparently, it was quite exciting. Spencer's team kicked some butt and won ten nothing. Spencer almost scored one of the goals. That was enough to get me off my butt and out to the second game. Besides, Tracey said she needed more batteries for the camera.

The second game was also quite exciting. All these soccer parents are turning into quite the fanatics. A few short years ago, they all started out as minivan drivers and shoelace tiers. As the soccer has improved, they've turned into rabid fans. Every good pass or scored goal evokes wild cheering. The missed opportunities are followed by cries of "Good try!" It's an electric atmosphere. I get a kick out of seeing Spencer out on the field being a kid and have about a thousand pictures of him more or less standing around on defense waiting for some action down at his end.

Each day of the tournament, the teams choose a couple of most valuable players. The coach had some nice things to say about the play of the entire team, making it difficult to choose any one that was truly outstanding. He awarded one of the prize MVP soccer balls to Spencer for doing well in circumstances that weren't always entirely in his favor. It brought a tear to my eye and smile to Spencer's face.

Sunday's games were against some tougher opponents. At half-time in the second game, I saw Spencer shifting his wool cap around on his clearly overheated little head. I brought him aside and suggested he didn't need to wear the hat and if he took it off, the other team would be afraid of him. He didn't say anything and just returned to his team. When he went out on the field in the second half, he had a kind of menacing grin on his face and he would look at the other team and rub his shiny head. It was cool.

A most valuable player indeed.

Nurk The All Powerful

We sat down for dinner tonight and Scupper had lost his mind. He kept diving under the dinner table pawing away, running between the chair legs and causing general mayhem.

I advised him in the most civil of tones that I thought his behavior was inappropriate. Which is to say, I barked at him in Klingon at a level just below the point at which he pees on the floor in mortal terror.

Then giggling revealed the true source of the mayhem.

Spencer had made an investment at the loonie store today. He bought himself some kind of small laser pointer. It projects a perfect target spot for Scupper to chase. With a flick of the wrist, Spencer can make a fifty-five pound dog bound fifteen feet across a room at high speed and crash in to the wall. Scupper positively wants to stun red spot with one mighty blow of the right paw and then chew it into individual photons, but it's too quick. It jumps on top of his paw before he can even stun it. On the ceiling, it's just plain unfair.

The effect on Spencer is no less dramatic. He giggles uncontrollably. We had dessert in the family room. Pumpkin pie on the coffee table with red laser spot? Not a good idea. Incorrect, Spencer. Do not lead your dog into temptation. Tracey came along and advised Spencer that it was time for his nabilone — more cisplatin was starting tomorrow. Was she crazy? Did she think the boy needed to giggle more? He took it.

As I was lying in our bed reading with Foster, Spencer was making trips back and forth into the room loading up his bag to take to the hospital tomorrow. "Nurk wants to bring his Gameboy." A moment later, "Nurk wants to bring his GameCube." Always in the third person.

"Who is Nurk, Spencer?" I asked.

"I am Nurk," he replied.

Nurk wanted to pack a television. Then Nurk wanted to pack the cable outlet so that he could get ALL the channels. Next thing you know, Nurk has a little red laser spot that tracks all the way up into the bedroom. "Look Noddy, Nupper has joined us." I screamed in Klingon, but I swear my heart wasn't in it.

Soon we all had new names bestowed on us by Nurk. Foster became Noster. Tracey became Nummy (she likes her new name). Scupper was Nupper, and I of course, was Noddy. As we were doing the final tuck in, the boys were shouting back and forth between their rooms. "I don't want to be Noster. I want to be Zoster."

"No, you have to be Noster. You must listen to me! I am Nurk, The All Powerful!"

I was all too happy to have Nurk The All Powerful safely tucked into bed. I was beginning to fear that I would look down at my crotch in mortal terror to find it illuminated by a little red laser spot with a fifty-five pound dog bounding forward determined to reduce it to individual photons.

Sparker Wants Mopcorn

These are words to please any parent whose kid hasn't eaten much of anything in the last two weeks. Last time Spencer was in good humor and being silly, he was Nurk, The All Powerful. The next day he was embarrassed for his nabilone-induced flight of fancy and took great offense at being called Nurk.

Then came the cisplatin. Then came the respiratory virus. Then came a little cough. Then came respiratory isolation in a room so dry we might as well have been living on aircraft for two weeks. There was an infection of his central line, the fevers, and the big gun antibiotics. Then came the diarrhea.

There went Steve's sanity. There went four kilograms of body weight. There went any chance of escape for at least another week. There went all humor.

The misery set in, and so it sits.

We were deemed unsuitable for the oncology ward. A biohazard. We all have the dry cough, So they threw us out to a new ward where we have to train the nurses.

Spencer's fever hits thirty-nine degrees with regularity. He just lies in bed, speaks only when spoken to, doesn't eat, and doesn't drink.

But today he felt like Yahtzee. We played many games. He ate a little bit of a cracker.

Tonight, he drank a glass of apple juice, and the nabilone is making him silly again. And hungry.

He said to Tracey, "Sparker wants mopcorn." When you hear words like these, you hang up the phone on your husband and you run for the microwave. And so she did.

I can't remember if I told her I love her, but I do.

Sparker ate the mopcorn. And the cheeseburger. And the pizza. And the macaroni. And a bunch of other stuff. He always seems to like to take it to the edge, just to the point where they want to stick a feeding hose down his nose and then a little voice inside him says, "Screw that idea!" And he eats and drinks.

There is something about hot melt glue and Nabilone that is compelling. He has spent the last two days gluing together Popsicle sticks. Now there are bird feeders with patios and tables and chairs, little fly-in retreats for the feathered set. One of them features a full set of Starbuck's logos and is eagerly awaited by its namesake coffee bar downstairs. The child life specialist has had to steal the inventories of craft sticks from all the other wards just to keep the factory going.

Somewhere inside, things have turned around. His blood cultures have come back negative for the nasty bug that had invaded his line. That's good, much better than going the other way. So the countdown begins. Seven more days of IV vancomycin and we will be free.

In the nether regions, things aren't going so well. The diarrhea continues. They called me yesterday. Could I bring them a stool sample?

"Do you need this collected in some kind of sterile fashion?" I asked.

"Oh no, that's not necessary," they said.

"So, just a regular collection will be fine?" I probed.

"Oh yes."

For clarification I asked, "Does it need to be a fresh one?"

"The fresher the better," they assured me.

"I'll see what I can do," I offered without committing.

I was so exhausted I nearly dropped it down the return slot at the Roger's Video store out of habit. They thought that was very funny when I told them about it at the clinic next door. I'm glad others are amused at the decay of my mind. It kind of makes it all worthwhile.

They phoned back a few hours later. No need to bring him in for his appointment. They had already made the diagnosis.

Scupper has roundworms.

I guess we haven't been giving him his monthly doses of Round Up or whatever we're supposed to administer. Too many damn medications. How can we remember them all? Now the nasty cling-ons are all making sense.

Ah well. Today was a CT scan, or half of one anyway. They didn't do his chest because the respiratory virus will give false positive readings. This was followed by an MIBG injection. Those scans are tomorrow and Thursday. Bone marrow biopsies next week. We'll see how this cancer thing is doing. I guess that's the whole point of this treatment exercise, even though it sometimes feels like it's just a test of character. For good measure, they're throwing in tests for heart, lungs, kidney, and hearing to see what unintended damage we've done and what headroom we have to do more.

Hard to believe we're only getting started.

Who's Counting?

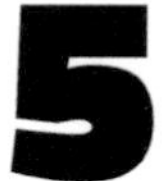: The number of deer that we saw on our way to the cabin this weekend.

26 hours: The time that Dirty Rotten Kitty lasted before Scupper managed to rip a hole in it and start pulling the stuffing out. I'm sure he loved his birthday present. He just loves things with his teeth.

2.6 kilometers: The distance we had walked on the Wild Pacific Trail before we got to the sign that read: "Warning: Cougar Sighted in the Area." But that was okay because it was starting to get dark so we couldn't see any cougars anyway.

90 minutes: The time that Foster squealed in delight as we stood on the overlook at Wickaninnish Beach watching the waves come in and hit the rocks throwing spray up and soaking the boys while huge breakers rolled in throwing massive logs into each other making thunder roll down the beach.

2000 miles: The distance some of the waves travel before they crash on the beach.

3: The number of black bears we saw munching on salmon in the rivers.

13 years: Time elapsed since I married Tracey on a stormy November day when the wind blew down trees blocking roads in Stanley Park where our reception was planned at the aquarium and she called to tell me that there might be a change of plans.

7: The estimated number of sea lions who were hauled out of the water just down from the cabin, based on the volume of their howling. Scupper is completely opposed to sea lions, even though he has never seen them.

104: Foster's count of the number of waterfalls we saw driving home when the skies opened up and fell down. A dozen of them were just falling off cliffs right onto the road.

8 feet: The length of Spencer's tubular knitting creation as he busied his hands while we travelled the highways and hung out in the cabin.

4: The number of ferry sailings you would have to wait when you show up at the terminal at 3:00 in the afternoon on a Sunday after a long weekend (which would mean an overnight snooze in the parking lot).

2: The actual number of sailings you have to wait when you tell them that waiting overnight is not an option because your son simply has to be back to start his chemotherapy at 8:00 in the morning.

60 knots: The apparent wind speed when a ferry travels at 20 knots into a gale that is gusting 40 knots.

15 degrees: How far you have to lean your body over to walk into a wind blowing at 60 knots.

6 minutes: The length of time it takes two boys to fall asleep after a long weekend in the rainforest on the West Coast of Vancouver Island.

The End Game

We're in the end game now. Down to two pawns and a king. The opponent still has a bishop and a knight. I won't say it looks hopeful, but it's not over yet.

I'd like to think it was just bad luck, but it's never just that, is it? There always has to be a failure in strategy.

I underestimated the opponent. Sometimes I think I am smarter and can relax a little bit. It's a fatal error. I let my guard down at the wrong moment, and it was almost over before I knew it.

It happened the other weekend at the cabin. Surely, Scupper could sleep upstairs? The rest of them were all for it. I couldn't see the problem with the logic. After all, it wasn't our house. There were no carpets, and he wasn't going to be allowed to sleep on the beds. There were no toys or Lego to chew, so what's the problem?

I gave in. The pawn moved forward and the bishop's path was clear.

Scupper, to his credit, was extraordinarily well behaved. He slept quietly beside the boys. He didn't come in and jump on me in the middle of the night. Didn't sneak up on me in the morning and stick a cold nose in my back or a wet tongue in my ear. He did his best imitation of a doormat.

I thought nothing of it. As far as I knew, the only thing that we had established was that the house rules were limited to the house, and vacations were a different matter.

It was three days later when the bishop slipped across the board and took my queen.

We were on our way upstairs to bed and Tracey put the little anti-dog gate to side and said, "Why doesn't Scupper come upstairs with us? He was so well behaved at the cabin." She smiled one of those heart-melting smiles, turned around, walked up the stairs and called, "Come on Scupper!"

He just slipped past me sort of melting into the wall as he went by, avoiding eye contact. I just stood there speechless at the bottom of the stairs. He's been sleeping upstairs ever since.

Spencer was just downstairs. He has a bone marrow biopsy tomorrow and was having a little trouble falling asleep so he came downstairs to warm himself a glass of milk. He wandered into the room and asked what I was doing. I said I was writing a story. He came over to the computer and saw the title "End Game" and read the first sentence. I had no choice but to sit him down and explain it all. Scupper and I are engaged in an epic battle and his mission is to displace me from my bed and forever relocate me to the couch downstairs.

Spencer had fallen under the spell of the black king long ago. He had no idea of the magnitude of the struggle. His solution was simple: "Why don't you just get a bigger bed?"

Checkmate.

Calibrating Love

I was tucking Foster in tonight. I was just about to head downstairs and so we wrapped things up with the usual ritual: "Goodnight Foster. I love you."

Foster: "I love you too."

Dad: "I love you three."

Foster: "I love you four."

Dad: "I love you nine."

Foster: "I love you ten."

Dad: "I love you infinity."

Foster: "I love you infinity and beyond!"

And that concluded the tuck. Or so I thought. But Foster went on. "I love you and Mom infinity and beyond. And I love Spencer a million. I love Scupper ten. I love Nanny and Papa nine."

"What about Grandpa?"

"I love Grandpa nine too. And if Grandma was still alive, I would love her nine, too. Is that right, Dad?"

"That sounds right to me, Foster."

Considering Grandma died when Foster was two months old, he maintains a fantastic sense of equity in the whole thing. Scupper gets a ten? No species hang-ups for six year olds. Oh well, at least it wasn't beyond infinity and beyond. Then I'm not sure what I'd have to do.

Christmas List

Tracey dropped me a note asking for stocking stuffer ideas and I responded as follows:

Okay sure. I have bottomless greed.

First, we'll start with the usual stuff. I would like peace on Earth and goodwill towards everyone. But these are often hard to find. You might want to see what you can find on E-Bay.

Right behind peace on Earth would come a decent 10" cabinet saw with a smooth fence system. But these are rather hard to fit in the stocking, and I'm loath to replace the ancient Rockwell Beaver that brings my Grandfather into the workshop on a regular basis.

So maybe some smaller items. Hugs from my boys. Nothing brings me greater joy. I love the fact that we have new couches with acres of seating area for everyone, and Spencer still likes to come and sit right on my lap even when he could have a reclining section of his own. So I'll have lots more hugs. Those are great.

The next one you might find kind of strange, but I would really like to have a Lulu Lemon Marathon running bra. This is the thing that I want most in the world because I understand that it would make you very happy, and what greater joy could there be than that? Besides, Scupper's never eaten one and they cause no nipple irritation. Unfortunately, they are as hard to find as goodwill to everyone, so let's move on.

I can always use socks and a new sweater. This is a horrifying statement because that's the kind of thing my Dad always says. I'm becoming an old fart that is difficult to buy for. Next thing you know, I'll be saying it doesn't really matter, it's all about the turkey.

You know, I always took Dad literally. I thought he was really a turkey fiend. I am sure he does like turkey, but I think maybe what he really means to say is that he just likes to have the family together and happy and that brings him the greatest joy at Christmas, but he is Dad, and he could never say that out loud. So we go on quietly believing that new socks and a drumstick bring him joy in life. No wonder he's smiling. I'll have new socks and a sweater.

Day -12

Right now, Spencer is doing great. We all enjoyed the holidays. We spent time with good friends and the boys enjoyed skiing and tubing and all kinds of fun. Spencer is in great shape. He has a ton of energy and is at an all-time high for body mass, but he still has cancer. The only clue is his bald head. So more treatment is in store.

Today Spencer is going into clinic for a checkup. Foster will also be at the hospital today doing an autologous blood donation. Tomorrow, Spencer will be admitted to hospital for intensive chemotherapy. Three or four days later, he will receive total body radiation over the course of several days. On or about the 12th of January, Foster will go into hospital and have bone marrow extracted from his hips. He'll get his own blood back at the same time and likely be discharged the same day or the day after. Spencer's bone marrow will be destroyed by the treatment and he will receive Foster's bone marrow through his IV line. How the little cells find their way into the cavities of his bones is a mystery. Then begins a long process of recovery.

The hope is that with the treatment and bone marrow transplant, and perhaps a couple of rounds of chemotherapy afterwards, Spencer will achieve remission. It is a very aggressive treatment and is very risky. If things go well, Spencer will remain in the bone marrow isolation unit until middle to late February. Friends and family are stepping in as house elves to feed and water Foster and let him out to pee and make sure that Scupper gets his meals and transport to and from school.

Today is Day -12. Day 0 is transplant day. That's how the medical people refer to it. If Spencer survives to Day 100, then he has survived his transplant.

If a Tree Falls in the Forest

If you expose your child to a lethal dose of radiation but then save them with fresh bone marrow, is it truly a lethal dose?

This was the strange question that went through my mind this morning as I took Spencer to the Cancer Agency for his first of six doses of total body radiation.

We almost didn't make it. I woke up and picked my watch off the shelf by my cot and noted what the time was. I felt well rested, but it was only 12:50 am. I almost rolled over and went back to sleep but decided to spin the watch around and have another look. It was 6:20 am when I looked at it the other way. Thoroughly confused and lacking any visual cues, I finally decided that my bladder was the best indicator and rolled out of bed. Always trust your bladder. We made it on time for the appointment.

Total body radiation is a bit of a different experience. The machine is not exactly like some of the other high tech gizmos we're familiar with that have the built-in DVD players with articulated flat panel video screens. It has more of a 1950s sci-fi feel about it. Spencer lays down on the floor on a rolling plywood platform. They line him up with marks and have little lead lung shields suspended in a frame above him. When they are satisfied that they have him positioned right, they drop sand bags all around his legs, torso and head. Then they slip an X-ray film underneath, turn on the Theratron 780C, expose the film, and make sure the little shields line up over his lungs. They didn't have it quite perfect the first go around and messed about with a ruler and felt pens moving things a few millimeters left and right until they were satisfied. They advised me not to worry; they deduct the X-ray exposures and make adjustments for the total dose. This was most comforting.

When I stepped outside to the operator's console, I was a little stunned. It was a panel with great big clunky backlit press button switches and little LED readouts. I felt certain that no Windows XP bug was somehow going to overexpose Spencer. "Wow, this is pretty much the best technology the 1970s has to offer, isn't it?" I asked the technicians. They weren't really sure whether it was that or the early '80s, but they reassured me that the Theratron 780C was the most accurate machine they had. It has its own onboard live cobalt and their treatment planning takes into account the half-life of the molecule. All much better than something that comes out of a linear accelerator.

Spencer lay motionless through the whole thing. I think it was out of comfort rather than terror. They would have had to strap me down.

So anyway, we are on Day -2. His chemotherapy is all done. Five more radiation treatments to go. Foster goes in early Wednesday morning and Spencer gets new bone marrow after his last radiation on Wednesday afternoon. The whole question is about as relevant as when the tree falls in the forest. Who cares? Just get the new bone marrow in.

Spencer is doing well. When he is not hooked up to an IV pole, he's been tearing around and has even gone outside to play in the snow. He's had to have baths twice a day because the chemo he is on works its way out through the skin and is a bit toxic so it would give him a rash if it's not washed away. Yikes.

Oh, and I Googled the Theratron 780C. The good news is that one of the first few links claimed, "Theratron 780C is accepted in the world as the gold standard in Cobalt therapy." The disturbing part was that when I clicked on the link it took me to the Morbai

Naraindas Budhrani Cancer Institute rather than John Hopkins or the Mayo Clinic.

Day −1 and Counting

They moved us out of the transplant room today. They are going to clean it out and put us back in it tomorrow.

The father's pre-transplant instincts return easily to me now. I wipe everything with alcohol. I touch nothing I don't have to. I take the less busy elevators. I open lever type doorknobs with my right butt cheek. Regular round doorknobs are more challenging. Given rubber pants, I would have a fighting chance with a two-cheek twister.

Foster checks in at 6:30 tomorrow. At 8:00 am they will suck his bone marrow out. Four hours in recovery and he'll be a free man. My guess is it won't be much fun no matter how many new stuffies he has.

Spencer has four more ambulance rides before he ends his relationship with the Theratron 780C. He has no fondness for the machine, and ambulance rides only sound glamorous when you don't have a tube down your nose and a barf basin under your chin.

Around 4:00 pm, they will hose him down with a pressure washer, insert him in the transplant room and give him his new bone marrow. I hope they keep it refrigerated. Seven hours is a long time to leave it lying around.

The nurse gave us hygiene instruction today, including personal hygiene. We must bathe regularly and wear gowns over regularly cleaned clothes, including clean underwear. I had to ask. They're not really going to check for skid marks. The underwear is on the honor system. I won't wipe the nurses with alcohol.

We established our first video link from transplant room to classroom today. There was no audio, so I keyboard chatted back and forth with Spencer's buddies. They even dragged Foster into the classroom so we could say hello. It was cool.

Tomorrow, the family will all be together under the same roof. It's not the right roof, but it's the same roof.

Day 0,+1, +2

When Spencer and I got on the ambulance yesterday morning, the dispatcher came on the radio and wished Spencer and Foster good luck for the day. Soon there were other ambulance drivers on the radio with their encouragement chiming in.

We had the radiation treatment. I let the team there know that they could read all about the Theratron 780C on Spencer's website. They were keen.

On the return trip, we swung by the ambulance dispatch station and picked up some hats and handshakes from the dispatcher. I'm not sure what Spencer and Tracey did the day before but they obviously made an impression on the ambulance service.

We did the mom and dad swap and I headed down to recovery with Foster. It may sound like I was the ever-present care giver, but it's all about boys being with their mom in their greatest moment of need. That's what drives everything. Thank goodness they didn't tear Tracey in half.

It didn't take long between apple juice sips in the recovery room and barf trays up on 3B before it was time for the swap back and the afternoon treatment.

I was nearly falling down with hunger by this point, but some angels were watching out for us. I had a vague recollection that Tracey mentioned there was some lasagna in the fridge. I bumped into my friend Sue in the parents' lounge on my way to pee. She asked if there was anything she could do. I mumbled something about lasagna, plates, and a microwave and ran back to rub Spencer's back. Soon the ambulance drivers arrived and I ran back to see about food. I looked in horror as Sue had cut into some other family's beautiful seafood lasagna rather than the Costco stuff that we had left over from Saturday. Then I looked at the label and it had our name on it. It was dropped off anonymously. I gobbled lasagna as they loaded Spencer on the stretcher.

We were finishing the last appointment forty minutes early after a variable schedule all week. They said they would try to get an ambulance to come early, but we would likely have to wait. I asked them to be sure to mention that it was Spencer looking for an ambulance. They laughed thinking that it wouldn't make much difference who was asking.

Two minutes later, there was a call from the ambulance service. Steve the dispatcher wanted to let me know that he was sorry, he was sending one from UBC Hospital, but it would still take a few minutes. He gave me a briefing on the twins who run it: two funny bald guys just like Spencer and me. They were great. Our host for the return trip even mentioned to Spencer that he had had a bone marrow transplant ten years ago, but not to worry: unlike him, Spencer's hair would grow back.

It was a long, tough day. Foster was ready to walk up and see Spencer an hour after surgery was done. The nurses weren't ready to let him go. They were worried about his hemoglobin, which was 109, and called Spencer's oncologist who performed the procedure to see what she wanted to do. She wasn't worried. Counts like that look fine to an oncologist, and she had firsthand knowledge of Foster's rather impressive marrow. 500 ml from a six-year-old!

When Foster was discharged, they let him have a wheelchair. Nanny was there in hers. He raced her through the hallways and won by a good margin. He rolled in the wheelchair, pleased to have his own medical special needs.

Spencer bathed and moved into the transplant room. Tracey, Spencer and Foster cuddled on the bed as the new bone marrow dripped in. It was nice to have the family all under one roof.

Foster is staying at home from school with Leanne and Uncle John. It's not necessarily because he needs to be, but sometimes it's just nice to get special treatment for a change.

We're all staying in touch by way of webcams. Spencer "goes" to school a couple of times a day. He says hello to his buddies and plays checkers and tic-tac-toe remotely. Scupper visits Spencer electronically. Mom or Dad can do electronic tucks from home. All very hygienic. No need to wipe with alcohol.

Day +4

We have now passed the easy part. Well, at least from Spencer's perspective. If you asked Foster, his hard work is done, except for the bits where he hardly ever gets to be with his whole family together. Now comes the rough stuff.

When Spencer had the treatment, it destroyed his bone marrow. The bone marrow is the stuff that produces all those blood cells: hemoglobin, platelets, and white blood cells. He had a bunch of those kicking around in his system. Now they are all being used up. The platelets and red blood cells are no big deal. He gets refill transfusions of those. It's those white blood cells that fight infections that are the problem. You can't get refills of white cells.

So Foster's bone marrow is busy finding its way to where it's supposed to be and then it will engraft. When it's done that, it will start to produce new blood cells and new bone marrow. That's going to take a while until everything is in full production.

In the meantime, we managed to take away Spencer's immune system, so he is in a bone marrow isolation room. It has positive pressure to keep the bugs from getting in. Brother Ron dropped some chili and other food for us today, so tonight the pressure might be a little higher than normal.

With no immune system, the bugs already in Spencer's system throw a party. He gets mucositis in his mouth and throat. That's kind of painful and nasty so he's on a continuous morphine drip.

Yesterday the fever started. Fevers are normal. They are also terrifying. We are terrified because of what it might be, but in a recalibrated cancer parent terrified kind of way. Which is about the same as how a normal parent reacts to their kid having a fever. You just look after them as best you can.

If I look on Spencer's IV pole at the moment, I see two IV pumps running four lines. Backing these up are two syringe pumps. There are six IV bags hanging. Finally, it's all rounded off by a feeding pump and a feedbag. It's so heavy that he has me push the pole down the hall when we get out for his bath.

I would list all the medications he is on, but I don't remember what they all are. There are four or five anti-nausea meds, a blood pressure med, one for his kidneys, maybe one for his liver, some antibiotics, morphine, and some other goodies to smooth the transition to his new marrow without having a bad negative reaction to it. He provides half time employment for one nurse around the clock. Which is an improvement over where he was. He used to have one dedicated for the first few days.

We are following the blood counts as we go. He's just about as low as he goes. We are deep in the valley and still going down. Hopefully, it's a pleasant valley, and a flash flood doesn't hit him. In a week or a month, he will begin the climb out again.

What's it like in the valley? Well, let's just say Spencer hasn't quite felt himself. The good news is he seems to have the nausea controlled. That's allowed him to feel better than he did at Day 0 to Day 3, so he's been playing cards and on his computer playing Neopets and exchanging the odd message with his friends. Things are a lot better than they could otherwise be. He says a few words now and then. He still walks to the tub room under his own steam.

We're doing okay, and Tracey has taken up watercolours. She painted an awesome picture of Scupper. I guess she has moved beyond the knitting craze. Busy hands are good for the mind.

Day 8

We'll drop the + designation. There seems to be little risk of confusing today with Day –8. On Day –8, I think Spencer was busy slapping the tongue of the wooly watercoloured wonder. Today he only managed a glance out the window at the beast before rolling over and going back to sleep.

Will and Sarah's dog Boston is now a certified therapy dog. Children's Hospital doesn't allow therapy dogs, and I'm not sure why. Since they're not allowed anyway, we saw no reason why Scupper would need to be certified, so I just walked him into the hospital.

There is a funny thing that happens when you do something outrageous like bring your dog into the hospital. He becomes invisible. It is obvious that he is a dog, and an energetic one at that, but if nobody sees him, then they don't have to deal with it. A crazy bald guy walking his dog through the hospital is not somebody you want to deal with if you don't have to. Even in the elevator when Scupper was dancing around, people just pretended not to notice. This suited me fine.

We walked him in through the back door of the oncology ward and out the parent's lounge onto the patio by Spencer's window. Spencer saw him, but wasn't really feeling well enough to care. Earlier in the day, the thought of seeing Scupper brought the first smile to his face that we have seen in a week. Timing is everything.

Foster came with me and Scupper to the hospital this afternoon. He had a follow-up blood test to make sure his hemoglobin had recovered from the bone marrow surgery. We don't need to know the results; we can accurately estimate hemoglobin levels by observation at this stage in the game. Foster has no worries there.

The visit was good. It's tough for Foster to see Spencer when he is not feeling well, but by the end of the visit Spencer was sitting up and playing cards and asking Foster, "Why are you wearing my shoes?"

Today was a tough day. Spencer barfed up his NG tube. The NG tube is how he gets all his "food" and oral medications. His throat is in rough shape so they don't want to put a new one in for three or four days, which suits Spencer fine. With the tube in, he hardly talks at all, and having a new one put in ranks among the most unpleasant of activities for Spencer. He would prefer a bone marrow biopsy to an NG tube insertion.

Unfortunately, with no tube, Spencer still has a few medications that he must now swallow. Swallowing is something you take for granted until you have mucositis. It took him three hits from his morphine pump to get down one pill tonight. It took a two-hour break and another three hits of morphine to get the second one down.

We'll take it one day at a time, sometimes an hour at a time. I have a feeling Scupper will be back. I tell the night staff that the rumors of us having a dog in the hospital are as outrageous as the claims that we were drinking ice wine with friends in the playroom the other week (by the way, a 50 cc syringe full of air with a long needle makes an excellent substitute for a corkscrew).

Sleepy Reader

I like routine these days. Routine is the crutch I use to prop up my mental shortfalls. When all is routine, I don't have to think about things. If I have to think, then my mind gets full and something has to fall out, and you never know what it might be. That's when bad things happen like you forget to put on your underwear or something.

So anyway, last night I was looking at the fridge and there was this note on it: "Wednesday is sleepy reader morning at school. Bring PJs, a stuffy and books to read." In my entire life experience, I have never encountered sleepy reader morning.

This was not routine.

I had a bad feeling. I would need Foster to help me through this. Which reminded me: where the heck was he anyway? Was I supposed to pick him up or was Shannon going to drop him off? He is with Shannon, right? Sure enough, he was and he arrived a short while later.

I asked him about Sleepy Reader morning. "Is this tomorrow or did it happen last Wednesday?" It was tomorrow. It was for the first half hour of school. "And are you supposed to wear your pajamas to school?"

"Yup."

"And do you wear them all day?"

"Uh-huh. And we are also allowed to bring a brother or sister or dad or somebody along if we want." He said it in such a way that left the door open, but it was clear that he wanted me to go.

"Do you want me to go with you?"

"Sure."

"And am I supposed to wear my pajamas too?"

"If you want. You don't have to."

Damned if I was going to let all the other kids' dads come in their pajamas while my Foster sat in the corner and read all by himself. I was up for it, but I had a dozen other questions. Who's reading, you or me? What books are we supposed to bring? French or English? What's this other note that says pack shorts and T-shirt for soccer practice? We had it all worked out. A fine plan was in place. As an added bonus, since we were going to skip daycare, we could sleep an extra hour.

Or, as it turned out, an hour and a half. Whoops.

That put a little pressure on the morning, but thank goodness for planning. Then Foster reminded me that I had to make lunch. Lori called wondering why he wasn't at daycare. Foster decided on sushi for lunch since it was already made in the fridge, which meant we had to figure out how to keep it refrigerated until lunch-time. I abandoned my luxurious plans to make coffee to bring in my Tim Horton's mug so I wouldn't be the sleepy reader. It was hectic, but it was a triumph. We arrived at school on time. Foster was in his PJs and a robe and we even remembered a teddy bear. I wore my slippers and a robe. But wait a minute, where were the other dads in their pajamas? Oh well. We read for half an hour and had good fun, and off I went to work.

I was brilliant; I even remembered the shorts and T-shirt to drop off at daycare, but I did forget the coffee mug. Better swing home and get it — can't bring those paper cups into the transplant room.

When I arrived at home, Scupper gave me a strange look. That one where his head is ducked down and he's done something bad, but it's up to me to figure out what it is. Damn him. I didn't have time for this. And then I saw it, the ever so slight indentation in the laundry pile on the couch that I intended to fold and put away, but never really got around to. Still warm. He understands "don't go on the couch" but he adds his own little dog qualifier "when the humans are home".

I grabbed my coffee cup and ran. I called Tracey just as I was getting close to work about forty-five minutes later. She had good news. Spencer has a white blood cell count today. Yes! Then she asked me about Sleepy Reader morning and I shared the tale of my triumphant fatherly deeds. She was clearly impressed.

"Did you bring him a coat?"

"Well, um. Yes. Sort of. Technically a housecoat."

"But it will rain this afternoon and they send them outside at lunch time." Oops.

"Did you pack a lunch?" "Of course. Foster decided to have sushi for lunch. We packed it in ice."

"Did you pack soya sauce or something for him to dip it in?" Oops.

"Did you remember to pack his soccer gear and take it to daycare?"

"Of course I remembered it. I have it right here beside me in the car." Oops.

Okay, so I nailed the Sleepy Reader part. So what if I missed a few of the details? When Foster spends the afternoon freezing as his pajamas dry out enough for him to go and be embarrassed playing soccer in them, I'm sure he won't remember it. He'll just think back to the warm moments we spent reading together, right?

Not likely. So Tracey made a few phone calls and dear friend Leila picked up some shorts, a T-shirt, and jacket and dropped them at the school along with a sandwich. Looking forward to a routine night tonight.

Day 18 - Trapped

There is not much in the way of news on Day 18. No news is generally good news. But it was not a day entirely devoid of news.

Today Spencer has an ANC, which is absolute neutrophil count. Neutrophils, for the uninitiated, are motile, short-lived polymorphonuclear leucocytes with a multi-lobed nucleus and a cytoplasm filled with numerous minute granules. With an ANC of 0.32, he has about 320 of these chiefs of the phagocytic leukocytes kicking around in a cubic millimeter of blood. At least that's my understanding.

In practical terms, it means the boy is starting to build up his immune system. Now, he's nowhere near strong enough to withstand the bacteriological onslaught of a Scupper fart, so the woolly beast has been visiting regularly on the patio outside Spencer's window.

There has been a small problem. On Friday, Foster, Scupper and I made our way up from the parkade through the elevators, down the hallways, through the tiniest corner of 3B into the parent lounge on our way to the patio.

Unfortunately, the door was locked. We were trapped. The only path to the patio is all the way across the ward by the nurses' station and out the back door near the playroom. We turned on our cloaking device and walked through, trying not to draw any attention to ourselves. Well, except for Scupper. He makes a career out of drawing attention to himself. But we escaped undetected but for a few nurses who I later convinced were hallucinating at the end of a long shift.

Spencer enjoyed seeing Scupper. We enjoyed seeing Spencer smile, and he's been doing a lot more of that lately. With the white blood cells has come a clearing of the mucositis, a huge reduction in pain, and a much greater capacity for enjoying things.

Saturday we left Foster, Spencer, and the GameCube alone with Uncle Ron while Tracey and I went to a movie. Date night with no medical intervention! It was wonderful.

Anyway, one of the first things that this new immune system wants to do is get rid of all the stuff that doesn't belong. Since the frame of reference is basically Foster, it pretty much figures that all of Spencer doesn't belong. It's called graft versus host disease. In its mild form, you get a bit of a skin rash here or there. In its severe form, it'll toss out your liver. Right now, Spencer has a few little rashy areas and Tracey and I have a new threat to keep our anxiety level constant. This is normal and expected and to some degree, desirable. They are also looking for a little graft versus tumor effect as well.

So all is well. We're starting to see a day or two ahead instead of an hour or two. But one day at a time…

Day 20 - Trust

Trust is an important thing. One of the fundamentals, really.

When our trust is violated, we slide into an uncomfortable world where things aren't as they should be. What we have come to depend on we can no longer. It's one thing for adults with their wary skepticism to lose trust, but quite another for a child.

I thought he might have lost his trust yesterday. His nurse came to reinsert the NG tube. He might as well have asked if it was okay to reach in and rip out Spencer's tonsils. Let me assure you that Spencer still has plenty of fighting spirit. I think the screams helped to keep his throat open while the tube went down, but in the end, it was just something that had to be done. No lies. No deception. Just a bit of unpleasant nastiness. Trust remained intact.

It's been a tough couple of days for Spencer. He's not quite feeling himself. His counts dipped a bit yesterday after an impressive rise the day before. We thought we were climbing out of the valley but met with a little ridge on the way up.

The doctors thought he might have had a fungal infection. An ultrasound was done and ophthalmologists were consulted, but in the end, no fungus. No more of the anti-fungal amphotericin, or "shake and bake" as the nurses call it. Good news.

Our little room on 3B has become quite a detox centre. The drugs are being reduced one by one. Today he is finished with morphine. Cold turkey was proven to be a really bad idea, so they ramped it down over several days. TPN will wrap up tomorrow, and they are going to take him off his blood pressure meds.

There's so much going on in his little body, it's no wonder he hasn't felt himself. The whole thing is an elaborate chemical balance and when one thing changes, the balance shifts and things need to be readjusted. Two steps forward, one step back.

The low-grade fevers continue, peaking every afternoon. It's hard to tell on the difficult climb when any of the loose boulders might break away and sweep him back to the bottom of the valley where the flood waters rage, but slowly he climbs with sure footing.

Enough poetry. Trust is the issue. His farts have let him down. He can no longer depend on them. They are untrustworthy.

We are burning through our supply of pajama bottoms and I have learned to change a bottom sheet in two minutes without Spencer's feet touching the floor or powering down the GameCube. Skills I hope to idle once trust is restored.

Day 22

Years from now, I will be in therapy working through my issues and trying to sort out why I have a fixation with skid marks, farts, and poo. For now, I'm content that I don't spend the day staring at the wall mumbling incoherently, and I can accept that I have issues that are unresolved.

While we are on the subject, Spencer has come to trust his farts. That is a beautiful thing because I forgot to take the laundry home yesterday and we would be fresh out of pajama bottoms by now if the trend continued. There is no recycling of pajamas with skid marks. His ANC is up to 0.5, and tomorrow he goes onto step-down isolation, which means he will be free from his room and allowed to go to the playroom for the first time in twenty-five days or so.

Today we were advised to get our house in order. Spencer will probably be coming home within a week or so. The house elves will be out in full force with rubber gloves and disinfectant on Sunday. Won't you, house elves? I can't think that far ahead. It was only a few days ago that I was thinking our next destination could be the ICU.

Today we were advised to get our dog in order. Scupper has to get a clean bill of health. The recommendations were very specific. There are four things they are testing for. I have no idea what they are. I only remember my instructions, which were very specific.

Saturday morning, Scupper has a veterinary appointment at 11:00 am. There is nothing terribly memorable about an eleven o'clock visit to the vet. No, the memorable part is that I must collect a stool sample. Not only do they want a stool sample, but also it has to be a fresh one, within two hours of his appointment. Oh yes, and I have to get him to drink a bowl of special broth. Scupper eats coffee tables, he doesn't drink broth, and we have never worked on pooping on command. So Saturday morning should be interesting and memorable. I'll be sure to write.

In the meantime, we've been very busy. I was given a shopping list today, which included double strand 24 gauge wire, a 3 Volt dc motor, an electric buzzer, wire cutters, D cell batteries, popsicle sticks, glue, and an empty two litre pop bottle. I'm not entirely clear on what is intended, but I'm sure Spencer isn't allowed any fissionable material in his isolation room so we should be okay.

Today was a good day. There has been no evidence of skid marks, farts, or poo, so I think I might be over my issues. Oops. Except Spencer is just asking for the commode. Gotta run.

Day Something-or-Other

They took them away today. Our houseplants.

If the truth were known, we didn't really deserve them anyway. It was a case of neglect. Not wilfully, just regular every-day ordinary neglect. These were only the ones that survived; the others we had already killed long ago. If you are a houseplant in the Dolling household, your life is destined to be a parched hell. It was just as well that the house elves took the houseplants away. If they get watered only once in the next two months, our plants are in a better place.

Some other things left our house today too. Every known bit of dust or lingering mould buried away in any corner or cupboard is now gone or slowly being killed by a diluted bleach solution. Unfortunately, I had to be with Spencer at the hospital and couldn't help with all the household cleaning, though I did consult by telephone when a rag hiding in the bottom of a bucket found its way down the toilet. Uncle John tried to convince me that it was a design flaw and not operator error. I'm not sure what was poorly designed, the rag, the toilet, the bucket, or the water. I hold operator error open as a possibility. An hour's work with my plumbing snake apparently dealt with the problem, or at least pushed it far enough down the pipe that when the toilet backs up two days from now, I will have forgotten the event and blame it on Scupper.

The inside of our heating ducts are also sparkling. At least I think they are. The nice man came on Saturday, wandered around, and gave me a quote for $385. I told him he was freakin' nuts as we had them cleaned a half dozen times before for less than half that amount. I called Tracey at the hospital. She advised me that we had never had them cleaned before because the quote was about $400 to have it done. I told the nice man to go ahead. It's a clever business. They drag in a really noisy machine and park it in the family room. Other hoses run out to the truck where a noisy compressor chugs away. They seal off all the heat registers and then go to work on them one by one. It's so noisy you can't stand to be in the same room. For all I know he sat and read a book for three hours and the machine's only purpose is to impress the homeowners. I never crawled inside the ducts to see if they are clean.

Scupper and I went to the vet on Saturday. There was a little confusion. He doesn't drink the broth. The broth is for culturing the specimens. I was impressed to learn that some of his specimens will travel as far as a lab in Edmonton. I was really impressed to learn that it costs $265 if you really want to have your dog's poo thoroughly checked out. When I gasped for breath they suggested, "Oh we better give Scupper another treat." This got him excited. He put his paws up on the counter and tried to sign the MasterCard invoice. Then he started knocking things off the counter. I think he was looking for $265 worth of treats. He does it all with a certain charm. He trashed the place, but left them smiling.

Tracey and I went out to a party last night for a close friend's fortieth birthday. It was high-end affair at a downtown hotel. They served real food on real plates with metal cutlery! Wine in stemware, not paper cups and cocktails with ice cubes. It was amazing. A wonderful time. On the way back to the hospital, I called the nursing station and asked them to let Uncle John know that we weren't coming back. We had learned to enjoy the good life and planned to catch the first available flight. The route to the airport goes right past Children's Hospital. We turned left, but the fantasy lived for at least twenty blocks.

Meanwhile back on 3B, Spencer continues to slowly improve. They are slowly taking him off all IV medications and stick them down his NG tube. He is interested in meals conceptually, though when they arrive, the reality is different.

A month is a long time to go without eating or drinking. It will take some getting used to. His counts are up and down but the trend is in the right direction. With any luck at all, they will pass the magic threshold, we will have good news from a lab in Edmonton, and a boy and his dog will be reunited under the same roof some time later this week.

Day 27

Tracey visits the pharmacist. The list is long. Magnesium, hydroxyzine, nabilone, ranitidine, cyclosporin, ondansetron, Gravol, Benadryl and Maxeran. The pharmacist felt compelled to warn of the side effects. "This one will make him drowsy. This one will make him drowsy. This one will make him very drowsy... Oh my God you're not going to give all of these to him at the same time are you?" Tracey nodded. "There is very little likelihood that he will remain conscious." Tracey smiled.

Meanwhile back in the room, the "over-drugged" boy is bouncing around on the bed. The nurse suggested I give him his four o'clock ondansetron before we go. I have no idea what to do with the NG tube. It's been a couple of years, but it wasn't a problem. Spencer showed me what to do. As he was forcing the air out of a flush syringe, he said to me, "You have to get rid of these little bubbles. They make you fart."

Seventeen loads of stuff down to the car later and we were ready to go. I never really thought I would be able to live in Shaughnessy among the multimillion-dollar mansions and have a staff to care for my family. After spending another month in the neighborhood, I have to say it's highly overrated. I much prefer our little hovel in the suburbs, even if we have to cook our own meals and wash our own sheets. I was happy to move out, though next time I think I'll hire professional movers.

So boy and dog were reunited. I was a little afraid that Scupper would think the NG tube was a toy to tug on, but it wasn't a problem. We have agreed that when it's time for the tube to come out, the easiest approach will be to tie it to Scupper's collar and throw a tennis ball. Spencer says Scupper has dog breath. I'm not surprised. He is a dog, and I didn't brush his teeth. That didn't seem to stop Spencer from calling him every ten minutes to come over and scratch him behind the ears.

Now everyone is heading for the beds. None of them have rails. None of them fold up. And I'm not entirely sure anyone will want to get out of them in the morning.

Dear Valentine

We're doing this for the twenty-fifth time. We ought to have it down by now.

Goodness knows there is a vast pallet of commercial sentiments to draw from. A dozen roses never goes wrong, but they are on the forbidden list this year. Another potentially toxic source of fungal invaders.

But that doesn't matter. Some fresh homemade pasta, a chilled bottle of chardonnay, steamed asparagus, a large Dungeness crab, candles, and some nice background music go a long, long way. A little odd that the most uplifting moment comes with the words, "Mom, can I have some more pasta?"

When I sit here enjoying the last of the wine as you give Spencer a bath in Aveeno to soothe his itching, I can't help but think that the proper way to do this is anchored in a quiet cove watching the sunset, listening to some wonderful music, and waiting for the evening dew and sky full of stars serving as background for the falling meteors. Chips of ice from the block, a glass of Bailey's, and a sleeping bag to cuddle in and ward off the dew.

But that's not our reality right now. Ours is the crushing weight of the day-to-day existence of clinic visits, endless medications, and a struggle just to get through the day. It's wearing a procedure mask and sleeping apart so that you don't get the same cold I have that would keep you apart from Spencer. It is scans and treatment and the horror of what might be.

Yet I feel little of the weight. As Spencer barfs up his NG tube and you phone the oncologist on call to find out what to do about the cyclosporine that lies in a puddle on the dining room table, I don't feel misery and sadness for what we have given up.

Instead, I feel a sense of wonder. For under everything is a solid foundation of love between you and me. That's what gives me strength. Sure, the romantic side is a little rusty. It's hard to find a baby sitter skilled in the medical arts and harder still to forget whatever it is we are escaping from, but I know these things will pass.

What endures is the warmth from your smile and the sense when you lay in my arms that everything is right with the world. That is as stronger now than it was twenty-five years ago. You are strength and beauty and wonder and love. So what can Hallmark, Purdy's or FTD add to that?

Don't get me wrong; I'm not an idiot. I realize that no medical ban on roses or any public proclamation of my love for you are going to get me off the hook. Tomorrow on the way home from work, I'll stop in and pick up some diamonds or other biologically inert material suitable for the occasion. Failing that, I'll just have to dip you in chocolate and lick it all off. Whatever it takes.

I love you.

Day 46

"Can't wait until my next set of scans."

"Why is that, Spencer?" Tracey asked.

"Because I don't think they are going to find anything."

So said the boy as they drove from the clinic to school. Yes, school. His doctor sent him on Friday. She saw him in the clinic finishing up his board game / circulatory system diagram / science project thingy and suggested that since he was doing so well, he might as well go into school for a little while and hand it in. So he did.

It's not as though he has been trapped at home. Earlier in the week he was at a radio station taping a commercial for the upcoming "Balding for Dollars" fundraising campaign. Spencer and I are poster boys this year. I'm going to have to grow some hair in a hurry or we won't be able to "shave for the brave."

Things have been going all right. In fact, they have been going so well that Tracey and I went out for date night. Our friends Bob and Sue took us out for dinner and a Pat Metheny concert. It was wonderful.

At dinner, Bob shared with us the heart-warming story of a Portuguese Water Dog that they had met. Some friends were looking after it and brought it along for New Year's Eve dinner. She was an eight-year-old black and white who was well behaved and just curled up at their feet. I'm not used to heart-warming stories about well-behaved Portuguese Water Dogs at dinner parties, so I found this a little surprising.

Then the story unwound as it should. They let the dog out and it ran away. Instead of enjoying lobsters, they spent most of the evening chasing this dog around the woods. They didn't find it until the next day when it was discovered at its own house whimpering in the driveway. "Yeah, that Roxie was a real piece of work."

Roxie? Scupper's mother is Roxie. I suppose there could be dozens of eight-year-old black and white females named Roxie who live in that part of town. Surely, this badly behaved animal couldn't be any relation to our Scupper. It hardly seems possible, but stranger things have happened.

We spent the rest of the weekend going to soccer games, lunching with grandparents outdoors in the sunshine, running Scupper on the beach, and hanging out with friends.

Life is trending back to normal. At least I think it is. I don't really remember what normal is. Which is nice, because that way I can pretend everything is normal and I won't be able to detect the difference. I do the same thing with my sanity.

Fifty-four days to go.

Hell in Little Pixels

I hate scan week. It's even worse when the week is spread out over ten days. Today was CT, echo, and bone scan. We still have bone marrow biopsies and MIBG to go. I think it all wraps up sometime around the middle of next week.

Anticipation brings out the manic-depressive in me. Early last week, I was convinced life was going well and it was finally time to move ahead with my midlife crisis: a Beneteau 34. I constructed an elaborate financial rationale and managed to convince Tracey, in my own mind, that we could afford it.

By the end of the week, I was convinced that we should sell the house, quit our jobs, and move up the coast to perform subsistence carpentry and dental hygiene in a mortgage-free environment where perhaps non-functioning brains would go unnoticed.

But reality is different. Reality is scans. This is perhaps the single most terrifying thing a parent can do: Just watch the screen and imagine hell in little pixels. You want to know, but the last thing you want to do is find out. Couldn't we go lie on a beach in Mexico instead? That would be more fun than watching, and worse, waiting. It wouldn't be so bad, but once you've fired the big gun, you hope to see results.

Ah well, other than that, life is normal. Sort of.

Tracey's mom is going to have her fourth artificial hip put in on Thursday. Number two gave out after years of yeoman service. Number three is still good for sixty thousand miles. She is in terrible pain, though she would never admit it to us. We worry about her. Though she would be upset if she knew we were using up our precious worries on her behalf. So we don't tell her that we worry, and then she won't worry about us.

It's much better if everybody just tells everybody how much they love them. Then no more worries.

MIBG Results

We had the big meeting today to review Spencer's scan results.

Tracey was very optimistic based on her experience as an amateur radiologist and factoring reactions from the techs and people in clinic who were in the know, but not at liberty to say what they know.

Tracey is much smarter and more perceptive than I am. Dr. Pritchard says that Spencer's scans look very good. She is very happy. The MIBG looks remarkably clear. There is one spot near his upper spine that she wants to consider blasting with focal radiation. They are also looking at a couple of rounds of irinotecan (chemo) and starting him back on retinoic acid after that. This was the intended path if everything went well.

Of all the places we could be at right now, this is about as good as it gets.

I am still processing this new information. It is not what I was mentally prepared for. We are very pleased.

There is other good news. Dr. Pritchard asked if we were going to go out on the boat this weekend. We said no because of the threat of black mould in the thirty-seven-year-old boat. She suggested that indeed that is probably not a good idea. I asked if I could infer from that that her recommendation was that we buy a new boat. She said she would write a prescription. I will check to see if it is covered under our extended health care.

Brilliant Green

Well, it was a busy weekend. Tracey turned forty and I shaved my head bald, but that wasn't really my gift to her.

No, this year I went for romance. After replacing her belts a week or two ago, they were newly tensioned and did in the bearings on the water pump. So for Tracey: a new water pump. And because I have to take off the alternator and strip the car to bits to get at it, I might as well replace the power steering pump while I'm down there, since it didn't sound so good either. While I was digging away to get at the bits, I noticed the timing belt wasn't looking so good. So might as well throw in a new one.

I really had no idea what I was doing. That's the thing about repair manuals: everything can be done in eight simple steps (which reference another eight simple steps, and so on). It's quite seductive. I have greasy fingerprints on five separate chapters. I was convinced that I could rip out the transaxle and replace the constant velocity joints and put new oil seals in the engine if only I could dedicate the whole weekend to the job. But of course, there were more important things to do.

My hair came out a lovely shade of green. The same brilliant green you find in that little flash on the side of the head of the male mallard duck. So we were off to Children's to shave it off. After all, people had paid a couple of thousand dollars to have me do it.

The problem was, we didn't quite make it there. Spencer kind of lost his legs just as we were nearing the elevator for the parking garage. So Tracey got a wheelchair and we took the other elevator up to 3B instead. A little hydration for an hour or so and Spencer was reasonably ambulatory with a wheelchair assist. We went and Shaved for the Brave and then headed straight home with only a minor detour to try to find a timing belt.

Things didn't go exactly as planned. Spencer never really picked up. Saturday night, he was admitted to hospital, and four bolt heads broke off on the water pump housing. Not that I grade these two disasters on the same scale, you understand. Figuring out how to drill out the old hardened bolts, find new ones and a corresponding tap, and on a Sunday, and then re-tapping the housing is no mean feat. Whereas Children's is staffed with experts and fully supplied 24/7.

Tracey woke up to her forties in the hospital with Spencer. Rather than relaxing at home with dinner cooked for her, we had take-out in the hallway at 3B. Seems to me we had her birthday here three years ago when Spencer was diagnosed.

Foster and I got the car back together again, but they still haven't figured out what's up with Spencer. A virus? Last week's chemo? Not really sure. He has a low fever and some pain in his back so they'll keep an eye on him here again tonight and we will see what the plan is tomorrow.

Never a dull moment.

Why can't we have dull moments?

Reap What You Sow

It's a funny thing when you grow out of your sandbox. No longer content to move piles of sand around with the toy diggers, you do new things like dig down deep. Really deep. Past the sand until you are mining strange new rocks.

That's where Foster got to. He had me scared when he said he found "tiles" that were broken in little bits. I thought he had excavated and smashed up the drain tiles on the foundation of the house. Turns out, it was only a few bits of concrete, but he had to be within a foot or two of the house electrical service.

We decided that the sandbox had reached the end of its useful life. We talked about what to do, and I suggested we rip it out and extend the grass. Tracey thought we could plant it as a garden.

Then I shared the story of the peas. When I was a boy, I took some of the leftover pea seeds after my Dad had planted his vegetable garden. I planted them in two short rows at the end of one of Mom's flowerbeds. I did nothing further until the end of the summer when I picked them and entered them in the fall fair in the kids' vegetable category. I won first prize — the blue ribbon and a five-dollar cash prize. I didn't mention that there were no other kids in town who happened to grow peas that year. A prize is a prize, after all.

Once we reviewed the theory of inflation, Foster understood that this was like winning $50 today. He was inspired. Anything with a chance of a financial windfall is interesting to Foster, so we decided to turn the sandbox into a vegetable garden. We did the calculations and figured we would need about five cubic feet of soil. We agreed to go out and get soil and seeds next weekend.

Once Foster is inspired, there is no waiting. When I got home last night, he wanted to go out and get dirt. I had to think about it: wash the dishes or have a trip to Home Depot? It was a tough call, but I couldn't deny my son.

Our calculations were wonderful except that they now seem to sell soil measured in litres. We went with three big bags. On the way to the cashier, we happened to bump into seeds, so we picked up radishes, carrots, green onions, lettuce, and peppers. We managed to get the sandbox filled with dirt before bedtime. Tonight was my night at the hospital. Spencer is still struggling with the whole eating and drinking thing, but seems to be steadily improving. He was feeling up to a game of Risk. I stopped by the nurses' station and asked if they could give him some Gravol and nabilone and threaten him with an NG tube placement while I went down to get a coffee. I hate to lose, so I look for any cognitive or psychological advantage I can get. He was unshaken and crushed me in the first game. I was coming on strong in the second when he declared bedtime just as I was about to take Africa and Australia. Nine year olds just don't play fair.

We called home to say goodnight. Foster picked up the phone. Sure enough, he had planted his seeds. All of them. Enough seeds to fill ten sandboxes with lush vegetables. He has pretty much followed my lead and regards instructions on the package as useless verbiage for wussies who don't know what they are doing. I think I am going to have to find a fall fair where he can enter his potential prize-winning vegetables. There are going to be a lot of them. You reap what you sow.

Quiet Rage

There's a quiet rage that burns within me.

Okay, perhaps that's overly dramatic. Probably stolen from some literary type. It is quiet, and it certainly has rage-like characteristics. Sort of that borderline kind of rage that has relatively high fear content. It is within me because I haven't shared it with anyone. As for burning, well, it's not really burning, but it's definitely there. What the heck, we'll run with it.

There's a quiet rage that burns within me.

Eight days we've been here. Sure there has been day parole, but at night we must return to our cell. The offense seems minor: a bit of diarrhea, some electrolyte imbalance, perhaps not enough eating and drinking. Every day we are on the edge of going home, and every day the parole officer says another day or two.

Tracey bears up better than I do. Saturday afternoon she threw a party on the patio. We filled the baby bathtub with ice to put the drinks in. Uncle John delivered a barbecue. Lonnie gave us two magnificent salads and the hospital foundation contributed a few dozen smokies for grilling. It was good fun. After a while, the nurses ran out of patients on the inside and they came out to join us too.

One of the dads brought out his fold up cot to show me. He had found a solution to the folding chair "beds" and sagging roll-aways that are the lot in life for 3B parents. I wanted one for my cell. I went to Costco that very afternoon.

For two nights now, we have had dinner parties at home with friends over. Wonderful warm breezes under the shade of the big umbrella. And each night one of us returns with Spencer to serve our time.

But this is all just interesting information. It has nothing to do with my burning rage-fear. The hospital folks are nice, and Spencer has dropped three kilograms, so I know they're really just looking out for him. No, to find the source of the building lava dome, we must move closer to home. Right to the family room. The epicenter of my nemesis. The habitat of the woolly black beast.

Some time ago, you might recall, the boys and I built Tracey a coffee table of driftwood, beach artifacts and memories to replace the old coffee table that Scupper ate.

Early last Monday morning, Scupper was working out his plan for the day, figuring out just what he might do with himself while the rest of the family was away, and he hit upon an idea that was a stroke of evil genius. He decided not to nibble away at the salty legs of the coffee table. That would be too obvious. But if he got up on top of the coffee table and chewed away at the inside edges, there is no way he would be able to trace it back to him. After all, dogs aren't allowed on the coffee table. We would be sure to think it was space aliens and never accuse him.

He managed to tear off a two-foot long chunk revealing bright yellow cedar to contrast nicely with the weathered patina. On the north end, he chewed off a chunk of the inset seal bone. Funny how he left the dog's jaw on the south end untouched.

Monday night, Scupper and I had a little chat. I think it is safe to say that he has disabused himself of the notion that space aliens are a credible explanation for canine misadventure. All I need to do is point at the coffee table and he slinks off shamefully to hide in his box. I've won this one. I know I have. He will never touch the coffee table again.

So off I go to sleep, bedding down on my comfy new cot. Another night in my cell, and the woolly black beast is lying at home comfortably snoozing away. In my bedroom. Next to Tracey.

There's a quiet rage that burns within me.

Wining

So do you want to come out to the garage when we're finished dinner and help me build the chairs?"

"Sure," said Spencer.

"But you'll have to be a little patient. I'm building them from plans and I don't really know what I'm doing so it will take a while to figure it out," I said.

"Dad, don't you find it a little unusual that when you have plans it slows you down, but other people would have to have plans to even build something in the first place?"

"Hmmm. Yes, I suppose it is a little strange."

We had Scupper to help. A few hours later, he was covered in a fine coat of red cedar dust and the chairs were complete and ready for a coat of stain.

It's a busy week. At least we keep busy. The go-kart was exercised though one of its drive pulleys split in two so the other one spins on any sort of incline. Mostly we parked it on the ridge at the park and fired off tennis ball rounds from the 60 mm air cannon for Scupper to retrieve. It's only a matter of time before we are arrested.

Speaking of law enforcement, the boys went to meet with Spencer's Cops for Cancer Buddy. They toured the Vancouver Police station, got to see inside a paddy wagon, drove at high speed in a police car with the lights on and came home with loads of goodies. We mustn't tell Will, but they liked the Vancouver tour better than Will's tour of the Burnaby RCMP detachment.

Tonight was the end of T-ball, the final game in the regular season. Foster ran the final leg on the round the bases relay and again assured victory for his team.

With the end of T-ball, we must prepare for hockey. Today, the boys went to the hockey store thingamajiggy and bought all the gear required for an ice hockey season except for a jersey and skates. Those will come later, I'm sure. What you have no way of knowing at this point, is that somewhere after writing about T-ball but before writing about hockey, a large quantity of wine went missing.

There is something wonderful about sitting on the patio and just chit chatting over a glass of wine, especially with the new chairs and the pergola whatchamacallit thingamajiggy overhead with the glowing candle lantern hangy bits. This week marked a watershed for us. Tracey loves Bin 65, and it comes in 1.5 litre bottles instead of the usual 750 ml, so I decided, what the hell? Let's go for the big bottles. Who are we fooling anyway? But alas, I digress. Foster now has the whole suit of hockey gear that hangs on a tree like a suit of medieval armor. He couldn't be happier. The gear was all used, except of course for the helmet, which you have to buy new. Interestingly, they discovered a new jock strap built into a set of ventilated boxer shorts with Velcro hangers for the hockey socks. But this is really far more information than you wanted, isn't it? Anyway, he wore the new jock to T-ball tonight and that was really nice because he didn't have to run all bow-legged. There was a bit of disappointment when I told him he couldn't sleep in it. Oh, now I've really shared more information than I should have.

Oh well. So now the MIBG scan is done. We just wait for the call.

I know what this is like from the parent's perspective. I wonder what it is like for the oncologist. Do they go out on their patios and drink large quantities of wine? I don't think this is easy on anybody, but if we stay busy, life's turning points can be lost amongst the trivia and somehow we can get through the next day.

Mini Donuts

We passed a milestone a while back. Foster now weighs more than Spencer, though he is three years younger. Not the sort of milestone you want to have for seven- and ten-year-old boys. Especially not when Foster doesn't have an ounce of fat on him.

But Spencer has been eating very well lately, and I thought my skinny boy might be regaining his position. So last night I weighed them.

Spencer: 59 pounds.

Foster: 60 pounds.

Scupper: 58 pounds.

A dead heat within measurement error. Today was the first day that Spencer was allowed to swim after having his central line removed last week. So guess what they did today? Yes, swimming.

Tonight we had free baseball tickets from the Starlight Foundation. Yes, free. So I paid for parking. The boys found the mini donut concession. And cotton candy. And more mini donuts. And soft drinks. By the end of the third inning, I was down forty-five dollars. By the fifth, I had to find the bank machine, so I treated myself to beer and peanuts and had plenty of cash left over for the boys to buy more mini donuts. They were gone a long time. The cashier was out of five-dollar bills and made them wait. They were rewarded with a free bag of mini donuts for their trouble. All sugar and cinnamon and toasty warm fresh out of the fryer melt in your mouth sort of mini donuts. They ate four dozen.

And the game was good, mostly because it is nice to sit on a summer evening in a ballpark without a central line. When your bony butt gets sore from the hard seat, Mom's knee is a comfy place to sit.

5-2 was the final score. Vancouver lost to Tri-Cities. I wish I knew which three cities. When we got home, it was way past bedtime, but not too late for me to demand an evaluation of the return on my investment. I made them get on the scales.

Spencer: 60.5 pounds.

Foster: 62 pounds.

Scupper: 59 pounds.

Where the hell did Scupper get the mini donuts?

Good to be Back Home

Snug Cove, Plumper Cove, Gibsons, Port Stalashen, Smuggler Cove, Secret Cove, Buccaneer Bay, Jedediah Island, Schooner Cove, Newcastle Island, Nanaimo, Telegraph Harbor, Ladysmith, Montague Harbor, Ganges and Otter Bay.

Scupper had a full woolly. On the docks, people would ask, "What is it?" Not, "What breed is your dog?" or ,"What kind of a dog is that?"

Just, "What is it?"

"It's a dog," I would explain.

Every day the boys swam. Well almost every day. Sometimes with wetsuits and sometimes with nothing. At Uncle Ernie's in Ladysmith, the water was seventy degrees, and the chicken was tasty.

Mostly the wind was with us and the sailing was good. There were dolphins, seals, otters, gulls and eagles, and on Jedediah, there were wild sheep left over from the Spaniards visits in the 1800s. They made Scupper look positively well groomed.

Then there were the prey species: Rainbow trout, rock cod, Dungeness crab, prawns. But no salmon. We decided to give them a break this year, or they decided to give us a break.

Midway through the trip as the boat grime built up, we checked in to the hotel at Schooner Cove for a night. They had electricity and hot and cold running water and huge beds with clean sheets.

Best of all, you could catch rock cod from the balcony on the second floor. Not that they encourage this, but there is no denying kids who have fishing rods.

Buccaneer Bay at low tide is like no place else on Earth, with warm tide pools and huge sandy beaches, and dogs playing volleyball with balloons.

Cracking crab in the cockpit, dipping in hot garlic butter, and throwing the shells overboard as the setting sun reflects off the greasy wine glass — that's living.

We never heard the words, "I'm bored." At least not from Spencer. Not with the new *Harry Potter* in his hands. We're not sure, but Foster might be growing gills.

Good as it was, it's nice to be home. Except for the fourteen loads of laundry. I mowed the lawn, I mowed Scupper, and I washed Tracey's car with the only soap that was handy: Hartz Groomer's Best Conditioning Shampoo.

Tomorrow, we'll try wearing shoes again.

Of Chickens and Goats

Well, we went for the PET scan and CT scan last week. The scan itself was a piece of cake. Just a hit of radioactive sugar and then I read *Harry Potter* aloud while Spencer lied motionless in the machine.

The scan has been reviewed, and the radiologist is scratching her head. Spencer is only the fourth kid in BC to have a PET scan and the only one with neuroblastoma. The problem with these things is that it is a bit like killing a chicken and spreading the entrails on a stone altar to predict if the crop will be good this year. It is all visible right there before you; you just need to have the right knowledge base to know what you are looking at.

The PET scan shows a couple of the spots that have been present for ages. Now the question is, what does it mean? The plan was to repeat bone scans and MIBG scans at the end of this month. Now they have decided they would like to move these scans up so that they at least correspond closely in time with the PET so they can cross-reference them and establish a baseline.

It's like killing a chicken this month and a goat next month and getting different results. Is it because goat entrails and chicken entrails tell a different story? Or have the gods intervened in between and the story has changed? So you have to kill a goat and a chicken together and then compare it to what happened when you killed the chicken at the last full moon.

Hmmm. I can see I headed down a very bad metaphor path.

Anyway, another radioactive injection next Tuesday. This will be followed by MIBG scans on Wednesday and Thursday, then different radioactive stuff on Friday morning with a bone scan immediately after. Then a meeting with Dr. Pritchard early the following week.

That ought to raise your anxiety level, but not nearly as much as it would be if you were a chicken or a goat.

Pray for a good crop.

More Desolation

We didn't have to kill anything.

But we did, of course.

There were a few things that we spared. At Savary Island, the big red jellyfish were the boys' intended targets, but somehow the water had cooled off by this late in the year. There were no jellyfish to be found, which was good. Murderous boys put their energy into building a cabin out of driftwood instead.

The prawns weren't so lucky. We caught many of them in and around Tenedos Bay, and the boys twisted their little heads off and we skewered their bodies for the barbecue. One was spared. Full of eggs, my friend Al decided that in the interest of conservation and setting a good example for the boys, it should be thrown back to the deep. It was a good lesson, but I still insisted that Al would eat one less than the rest of us. There is price for every lesson.

The big rock cod? Dead. Left to die in the bucket until we returned to the East Wind where we introduced it to a sharp fillet knife. Fillets for dinner. A head for the crab trap and the rest as halibut bait.

The halibut were somewhere else, however, or at least they choose to grace the hooks of fisherman smarter than us. In their place, dogfish: large mud sharks. At least five of them. We didn't kill them though. By the time we caught the third one, same size as the first two, we started to wonder if perhaps it wasn't a single specimen with a serial propensity for a painful elevator ride 200 feet to the surface. "Could they really be that stupid that they would bite the same hook over and over again?" Spencer asked.

"Please, Spencer," I cautioned, "don't call them stupid. Stupid is not a nice word. This dogfish is cognitively challenged."

"Could it really be that cognitively challenged that it would bite the same fish hook over and over again?" he asked.

"Spencer, you understand that by using a politically correct term like 'cognitively challenged' that you are really just attaching a new label to the same thing and over time it will come to have exactly the same meaning with all the same connotations and that you end up being just as politically incorrect but now you are doing it with a fancy five dollar word? Would you agree, Al?"

"Yes. Give me another chunk of bait. I want to catch another stupid dogfish."

We caught him a few more times and returned to East Wind as the sun was setting. While we were gone — much excitement. The cod head we converted to five Dungeness crab: 3 females and 2 undersized males. We threw them all back.

We're not really the killers that we think we are. We just like to believe that we are dangerous and manly with a hint of recklessness and a bit of a fishy odor. We think that Tracey and Sue find us irresistible that way, but I suspect they just like us to go away in the dinghy so they can enjoy some peace.

Finally, we killed a fine bottle of ice wine and about a pound of the delicious dark chocolate almond bark from the general store at Squirrel Cove. And so ended three days of death and mayhem with good friends in that little dream they call Desolation Sound. Okay, now I'm ready for fall.

RELAPSE

Re-lapse: 1) recurrence of disease 2) that period of time where the child and parent have been faking it so long they actually believe everything will still be okay 3) The stories of Spencer from age ten through age thirteen

Dick's Lumber

I'd never been there before. I guess it's because it's a long way from home, but it's only five minutes from my office. It's a manly man's lumberyard. I stopped in there at lunchtime yesterday. It's impressive. They have serious lumber, any kind you want. It's the kind of place you can drive around with a flatbed trailer and have them load a few thousand board feet of anything with massive forklifts. The office / retail store is brimming with people servicing the contractors who frequent the place. I walked up to the desk and requested a quote on rough sawn two by tens in red cedar. It was running a little less than four bucks a foot. I thanked the man and left.

I had no plan to return today, but plans change. So there I was, back at the desk, with the same guy as yesterday. I told him I wanted to buy some two by ten rough sawn cedar.

"What length?" he asked.

"Eight feet," I replied in my manly man Dick's Lumber customer voice.

"How many?"

"Uh, just one."

"Weren't you in here yesterday?" he asked.

I guess they don't have many customers who come in one day, request a quote and then spend another day thinking about it before committing to a thirty-dollar purchase. "Ya," I replied. Some of the manliness had left my voice at this point.

After determining that I didn't have an account, he sent me over to the cash desk and on to shipping with the yellow copy of my invoice. "Just pull it over here," the shipping coordinator gestured to the line of trucks outside, "and somebody will be out to give you a hand."

It's safe to say I was the only guy at Dick's today driving a Harvest Moon Beige VW convertible. I tried to look manly while I waited in line with the top down. Eventually the picker came and grabbed my invoice and figured out what he was looking for. "Let's see. Two by ten cedar." It was in a bay blocked by a truck. No room to get a large forklift in. Not that you need a forklift to get a single board, but when the bundle of eight footers is racked twelve feet off the ground, you need to bring down the whole stack. We waited for fifteen minutes while the picker made repeated radio calls for a "small machine" to the two by ten cedar. None came. Eventually the big truck moved and there was enough room for a "big machine" to come in. They lifted down the thousand pound stack of lumber and the picker chose a fine specimen for me.

I was able to load the entire board into Tracey's car without benefit of a forklift. I said my farewell to the picker: "I'm not sure my wife is going to appreciate me transporting lumber in her car."

"As long as it's your wife's car," he said, and I was on my way.

I spent the afternoon engaged in wood therapy, fashioning post caps to complete the fence. Therapy was required because this morning Spencer's oncologist let us know that the scans show new spots. New spots aren't good. I didn't even like the old spots. I definitely don't like the new spots. So it's a bone marrow biopsy, a new line, and some fresh chemo coming soon.

I think I'll go back to Dick's. Surely, they have something at Dick's that can fix this once and for all.

Windmill

Spencer had a five-day round of topless cyclone last week. At least that's what we call it out here on the west coast. I think on the Atlantic coast they must call it a semi-naked hurricane. Lay people would know it as chemotherapy. I think it went well. At least he kept eating all week and never barfed once. I hope it does some good against that cancer thing because it showed up in his bone marrow again for the first time in three years.

Spencer had hoped to get his school picture taken while he still had hair. The oncologist arranged for chemo to start a little later on Thursday so it could happen. Unfortunately, the teachers went out on strike for a couple of weeks and the schools were shut down, so no photos. But they go back tomorrow. I imagine the mediator made it clear to all parties that there were kids out there who wanted their pictures taken while they still had hair so they had better settle their differences. And so they did.

That's not to say there was two weeks without schoolwork. We completed a science project. It had to demonstrate simple machines and pulleys. Dads were allowed to help, so naturally we built a windmill with a drive shaft and pulley mechanism that can lift a hammer with the wind from a small fan. I asked Spencer what he would say when his teacher asked who built it. "Well, you did and I helped," he said.

"Really? Who cut the tower columns to length with the saw?" I asked.

"I did," he replied. "And who nailed the tower columns to the base?"

"Me."

"And who nailed the top part in place? And who went to the hobby store to buy the shaft and bearings? And who nailed the top part to the tower and the bearing blocks to the top part? And who cut the shaft to length with a hacksaw?"

"I did."

"And who sanded the winding drum on the lathe and drilled the hole down the center and cut it off from the waste block?"

"Me."

"Uh huh. And all I did was cut out the blades and make a few pulleys. So who really made the windmill?"

"I made the windmill, and you helped a little." And so it was.

Happy Halloween

It was against my better judgment. My better judgment ranks as only average judgment among the general population, which made it all the more troubling that we went ahead regardless.

The boys wanted to go with the Captain Underpants costume. Who was I to say no? Especially since this year, I wasn't the target.

That's not to say there wasn't a struggle. There was quite some discussion about where the tail would go. Foster suggested it should come out "the penis hole".

The boys grabbed Scupper and I worked on a pair of Foster's old underpants. Soon he was ready to go, except for the cape.

And then he went.

Bouncing all around the living room, nipping at his new underwear.

That was last week. Since then Spencer had a bad reaction to some platelets, spiked a fever and was incarcerated for having a body temperature 1.5 degrees above the average for the population.

Yesterday he was released on day parole. They didn't want to let him go. The new fellow suggested that releasing the boy with hemoglobin of eighty and platelets in the twenties was not a good idea. I didn't think keeping him shut in the hospital was a good idea and so I promised that I would not let him near any power tools or sharp objects and he wouldn't run any marathons. I promised to have him back by 6:00 for fresh hemo-goblins.

So we left the hospital. Soon the boys were at home in their element with sharp knives in hand carving away at pumpkins. The little pumpkins were fun, but when Tracey talked to neighbour Susan about a somewhat larger pumpkin, we were on our way to her dad's house to select one from the garden. We ended up with a smaller pumpkin, probably only 150 pounds. We loaded it up and headed home. Time for power tools.

All was set for Halloween, except for the incarceration thing. But with another transfusion of platelets, they released Spencer for good just in time for Halloween today. Foster hit the streets as an alien and Spencer dressed as the Grim Reeker — the electronic fart machine providing the soundtrack.

And Scupper? Well, it turns out that better judgement prevailed. He decided not to dress up and stayed home with me to howl at the doorbell.

Luxury Dog

The good folks at the Chateau Whistler decided our family deserved a free weekend in their luxury hotel. I'm not entirely sure why. I think they felt sorry for us because we have so little hair.

Now that I think about it, that probably was their bias.

As we were making plans, we had to think of Scupper. It's his birthday this weekend. Now, I don't usually think of Scupper and luxury hotels in the same synaptic firing sequence, but Tracey made inquiries. As it turned out, Scupper was more than welcome to come and stay at the Chateau Whistler, but because he has more hair than the rest of us combined, we had to pay $50 to bring him. What the hell was I thinking?

He wanders around every day in a black and harvest moon beige tuxedo. His formal wear grows on him. He fit right in at the Chateau Whistler. His little doggy bed, stainless water dish, and complimentary treats were all waiting for him on arrival. He settled in nicely, and he makes friends wherever he goes.

Saturday morning, the concierge said good morning to me. For Scupper it was, "Scupper, good morning. How are you? Happy birthday buddy!"

I locked him in the car. I couldn't find a coffee table in the hotel room, but I'm sure Scupper would have found something to destroy. The rest of us headed out to the ski rental shop.

A lot has changed since I last went skiing. We all rented gear. The new skis are shorter, wider and much more shapely than they used to be. It's all to make skiing easier for older, fatter, out of shape baby boomers. I was grateful for their efforts, though I would never confess to being old, fat, out of shape, or a baby boomer. I think I will throw away my old long skinny things that tower over my head. I'm not sure about my boots. I think they fit fine, but they are buried in the crawl space and I hate going down there because I am old, fat and lazy. The rentals were fine and everything was half price this early in the season.

Foster blew a ski just as he was getting on his first chairlift. That didn't seem to bother him. He managed to ski off on one ski and the next guy off brought Foster's ski with him. We got on the next high-speed quad chair headed for the top of the mountain. It's a long way to the top of Blackcomb, something like a mile of vertical.

Once we were up, we were committed, which isn't necessarily a very good idea. Ski school would have been a smarter idea, but we weren't sure if Spencer would hold up through a whole lesson. After he had fallen down twice in the first couple of minutes, he decided he didn't want to ski. Tracey and Foster carried on and I worked with Spencer a few feet at a time until we made our way down to the long flat green run that goes many miles down the mountain. Eventually Spencer started to enjoy it once he realized he was in control and it wasn't a "point your skis downhill and live a moment of terror until you crash" kind of thing. It is possible to turn and stop.

We ended the day after his legs ran out of steam, though not in a real convenient place. We could see the mid-mountain chair for downloading, but it was a long route to get there on blue and green runs. By this point Spencer was walking over a difficult bit with my poles while I carried his skis.

No sooner had I suggested that we could get there more quickly going straight down the black diamond route than he was off on a black diamond butt slide. I don't do black diamonds and definitely not without my poles while carrying extra skis. I did my best to keep up sliding on my butt. It wasn't long until we were back on the chair on our way to the village.

No training was required for the swimming pool, hot tubs and sauna. You dive in the water inside and swim under a wall to the outside pool. No need to get cold. When your head starts to freeze, you just duck under water for a bit. The boys loved it. We ate out at restaurants and had no chores to do.

Scupper wasn't too pleased that his welcome wasn't extended to the spa and restaurants, but he had fun overall. Sunday morning I woke up to him barking to get out the door. I dressed and took him down. We weren't ten feet out the door when he ducked into a squat beside the valet desk preparing to unload.

Yes, he's definitely a class act worthy of the finest hotels. He would never attempt to poop in the lobby.

Today was a start of a new round of chemo for Spencer, albeit a short one. His kidney function test from last week doesn't look so good, so it's off to the kidney specialist. There is no such thing as a real break.

The Truth of Fresh Baked Bread

There is no real deadline for such things. Somehow, this year we started out with transplant and just never got around to it. At some point this summer, I recognized that I was probably a little overdue, even though there is no deadline, so I started to take the Christmas lights down.

I removed one full string from the gutter on the back of the house and the next I left hanging half off, intending to move the ladder over the fence into the front yard to complete the work. Then at some point I noticed the fence was falling down. And sailing season set in. And, well, then came the granite and the cedar and the Christmas lights just stayed there.

The guilt persisted about to the point where the leaves fell off the trees. Then I realized I wasn't lazy, I was clever. I already had the jump on my neighbors. Those poor bastards would be struggling in the rain and cold clipping the lights onto their gutters and all I would need to do is put up one string and plug them in.

Well, they've been busy. Now the neighborhood is all lit up. But not my house. There's just one string to go, but now there is snow and ice and cold temperatures to deal with. I feel a deadline looming.

Scupper feels no such pressures. I'm not sure he prepares for anything. He just sort of lives life in the moment. The other day, for example, I seriously doubt if he woke up and decided he wanted to eat a half loaf of French bread and would take steps to make it so. He just happened to be in the car with Tracey and Spencer when they dropped in for groceries. When they stopped in at daycare to pick up Foster and left him alone in the car, the French bread just spoke to him and said, "Scupper, live for the moment. Feel no guilt. There are no consequences."

The French bread lied, of course, but when you live in the moment, you don't connect those screaming unhappy humans to anything that happened in the last moment. They're just plain irrational. French bread always speaks the truth.

Sometimes I Write

I never sit down at the keyboard and think, "Hmmm, I wonder what I can write that might make somebody laugh or cry or think profound thoughts," and then go about toiling away with ideas forming them into sentences and paragraphs until they're just right. For me, it doesn't work that way.

Things just kind of bounce around in my head and then somehow organize into a complete set of thoughts that just drops out of my brain onto the keyboard. Sometimes I think it is the result of internal thought pressure in my brain that exceeds the threshold and then some valve releases the moment they are organized into any kind of coherence that might be understood by fellow humans.

Even at this moment as my fingers are toiling away, I am not struggling as to what will come next. It is already fully formed and I just watch the words come up on the screen as some sort of validation of thoughts that have already been fully processed. I don't yet know how many paragraphs there will be or exactly what words I will use, but that will all become clear to me in a few minutes.

Sometimes what I write has three or four levels of meaning. Sometimes it's just plain silly and people are just used to scratching their heads and wondering what I'm really saying and read more into it than I ever intended. I get to marvel at the meaning that somebody else derives when my dog eats a loaf of bread. It's all good fun, generally.

But I'm not rattling along here in some sense of self-exploration or trying to convey to you what the writing process is for me so that you can gain insight into how my brain works. That might be interesting, but it's not where this is destined. No, I just share this with you so you will understand what follows. I want you to understand that this isn't something I necessarily control or even do consciously.

Today on the drive home, I had a writing moment. Well, two: this one and the one that preceded it. This one you'll fully grasp in a moment. The other one was a much more frightening experience. It left me staggered and shaking and in tears for the last half of the drive home. I had to pull over and park in the Home Depot lot for a while.

Often a bunch of thoughts rattle around in my brain that sometimes form a coherent whole, which I dare not put through the later keyboard process because I'm not sure how others might react to them. These are dark or strange thoughts that could be disturbing to others but quite happily exist in my brain all the time.

So today, what came fully formed in my brain was the darkest and most frightening thing that could have possibly formed. Disturbing, even for me. Fully formed and complete in every respect except for perhaps the final words formed into sentences and paragraphs.

Spencer's eulogy.

It was beautiful and powerful. A fitting tribute with meaning and clarity. Utterly moving and filled with joy and sadness and dignity and purpose. Something I dare not put to keyboard. We'll leave it at that. Hopefully, it fades and gradually loses shape and form, and it will become a dim memory of my greatest piece of writing that never was. I know it will not fall on this keyboard tonight.

Eating Dogs

When I arrived home tonight, the boys were already eating dinner. They had those hotdogs with the Pillsbury dough wrapped around them and baked. They were dipping them in ketchup. I love those hot dogs. I dip mine in mustard.

"Oh, are we having hot dogs?" I asked.

"The boys are having hot dogs; we're having basset fillets and baked vegetables," Tracey said.

I looked at Scupper. It's been a long time since I've been to Korea.

"Basset fillets? Like the dog?"

"Not basset. It's a fish: basa."

"Bass?" I asked. I know what a bass is.

"No, Basa," she explained.

Maybe it's like an Italian bass. I'm not sure what a basa looks like before it's filleted. Probably something ugly with a bad name that somebody in marketing got a hold of. It was a wonderful fish, beautifully prepared.

Anyway, I digress. Spencer is happily eating hot dogs because he didn't start chemo today. We are trying irinotecan again. Last time he had a very bad time with it from both ends. Kind of like Scupper the day I learned how to remove the carpeting from the cargo area of the Pathfinder and Tracey forever said goodbye to the serving spoon from the kitchen. So this time around, they know what to do and are hitting him with two days of a special antibiotic before they start. Hopefully this will be easier on him. The irinotecan, though hard on his gut, is apparently easy on the kidneys, so he starts Wednesday. And it's a good thing. Spencer is starting to get a little stubble of hair, and I hate to see him looking that way.

They are planning to admit him on Friday to finish the five day round over the weekend. If he is feeling okay, we'll get out on day parole. If he is having a rough time, they will be able to better control it in the hospital before he gets dehydrated and really sick like last go around.

Everybody is doing well. Spencer played the full game of soccer on Saturday and road hockey on Sunday. Foster had two rounds of ice hockey and a soccer game as well. I can't remember what else we did last weekend. Is it really only Monday?

Efficient Market Theory

There was a time when they funded the public education system decently. Now, I'm afraid, they aren't even adequately funding teacher pensions.

Today, Spencer's teacher instructed everyone in the class to each pick five stocks. They will follow them for a time and then the winner will be chosen. I suspect the real purpose is for Mr. Barabe to identify his best choice for a free financial advisor. It's a shame; he is a good man, they should really be properly funding his pension.

In any case, when I arrived home, there was much excitement. I was to help Spencer pick five stocks.

I didn't have the heart to tell him that his chances of winning the competition were equally good if he had Scupper choose them, so I did what I do best. I faked it.

We started with a review of portfolio theory. We discussed stock volatility, the tendency of all stocks in a sector to move together, the advantages and disadvantages of having a balanced portfolio, what makes a good company and how that is reflected in the stock price, why a company with a low price might be good investment, price / earnings ratios, efficient market theory and a number of related concepts. The frightening part was I think he got it all.

We set about putting together a written plan for his portfolio management. There were several key elements that he chose:

a. He chose a high-risk approach over a low risk approach because it's not his money and he wants to win the game even though he understands that it could put him in last place with the wrong luck.

b. He is willing to invest in companies he has never heard of because he recognizes he is a kid without much market exposure and doesn't want to limit his opportunities.

c. He rejects efficient market theory because he believes that there are scammers and market manipulators who move the price and their movements are not random.

d. He prefers to have a diversified portfolio over a sector specific one.

e. Finally, when asked whether he would like to choose stocks that have performed well recently or may have been underperforming but represent superior upside, he chose a mix of both.

With these somewhat conflicting guidelines, he decided to choose stocks from the financial, energy, minerals, retail, and communication sectors. We set about diving into the TSX website and reviewing the companies in the various sectors. Unfortunately, bedtime intervened, so he wasn't really able to do any in depth comparison of the companies. He did what many investors do: he pulled up a company in the sector and had a glance at the charts looking at performance over five years and the last three months. When he saw something he liked, he went with it, more or less following his guidelines. His five stocks were chosen.

Now back to Mr. Barabe. I think I shall have to sit down with Scupper and see if he can help with some selections for his portfolio. It will be a good test of the efficient market hypothesis.

Then again, Scupper might be an insider...

End of Season One

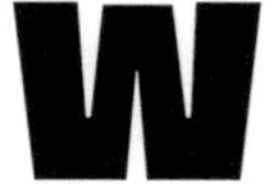e sometimes wonder what goes on inside our kids' heads.

This year Foster begged and pleaded to play hockey, but it was not high on our list of things to do. Of all the sports out there, why pick the one that costs a small fortune to play and forces you to get out of bed at five o'clock on weekend mornings? But it was his passion, so we relented. We are Canadian, after all.

All the other kids started playing hockey two years before him. I'm not sure Foster imagined starting out at the bottom and being one of the worst players on his team, but his coaches were all fantastic. They were dedicated to the kids having fun and learning skills. With encouragement and good coaching, Foster made excellent progress. He's now solidly in the middle of the pack. Given another year, I wouldn't doubt if he could become one of the top players if he put his mind to it. He's doing great.

So we were a little surprised when a month or two ago, Foster declared that he didn't want to play hockey next year. We always moan and groan about getting up early. Foster likes to please, so we shut our mouths. The dialogue changed from, "Shall we draw straws to see who has to get up at some ungodly hour tomorrow to take Foster to hockey?" to, "Hey, can I take Foster tomorrow? I wouldn't want to miss a game." We were much more positive. After all, if it's what he wants to do, we will support him.

I thought things had turned around. A couple of weeks ago they handed out the forms to register for next year. We asked Foster if he wanted to play. "I don't want to play hockey next year."

"Why not?"

"It gives me a headache."

A headache? That sounds like an excuse. Did I mention that Foster isn't just a developing player, but he happens to play on a team that has lots of development to do? That's code for "they hardly ever win a game." Maybe it's just a lot of work for little reward. But we kept probing. Tracey talked to the coaches to make sure that he was getting hydration. He stuck to his story. He didn't want to play hockey because it gives him a headache.

Then Tracey took him in to have his skates sharpened and brought his helmet along. She asked the folks at the hockey shop to check out the fit. They were shocked, "Who fit this helmet?"

"Ah, you did." Tracey explained as she watched them turn various shades of red. They went about adjusting the helmet, expanding it to the outer limit of its expansion range. It is still a bit tight, but quite a lot better. We decided to see how he felt after the final tournament.

The final tournament was interesting. Officially, they don't keep score, but kids aren't stupid. They can tell when they are outgunned by a ten to one margin. In one game, Foster was goalie. The Poco Red Devils appeared to be standing still as the team from Chilliwack skated circles around them and had three periods taking shots at Foster. He made spectacular saves, but a fair number, well maybe a huge number, made it past him. It had potential to be soul destroying. I had memories of a soccer game when one of the kids let in a couple of goals and then ran off into the woods to escape the humiliation. Poor Foster had nowhere to run. But in the end, the clock ran out and his team all dog piled on him as though he had just single-handedly won them the Stanley Cup.

The final verdict? No headaches. Foster discovered that hockey is fun and not just something you do for pain. He wants to play next year.

As for us adults? Well, I guess we should stop wondering what goes on inside our kids' heads while we are busy crushing their brains from the outside.

Another Normal Day

Today was an interesting day.

The first remarkable thing was traveling down the highway somewhere outside Nuremberg at 4:00 am in a taxi doing a little better than 180 km/h. I wasn't used to that, but I guess that is fairly normal in Germany. By the time I was in Amsterdam, my luggage had disappeared to the nether regions of the Netherlands. For reasons that only airlines will understand, it is cheaper by half to fly from Nuremberg to Amsterdam to Frankfurt to Vancouver than it is to just fly from Frankfurt to Vancouver. So by the time I made it back to Germany, I knew for sure it was going to be a long day.

Originally, I had planned to visit my friend Will in the hospital when I returned home. As luck would have it, Will is now in intensive care, and visitors are now limited to immediate family only. I was left with some free time, which was fortunate because as it turns out Spencer was admitted to hospital sometime between Amsterdam and Frankfurt. A little pain in the shoulder: nine out of ten on the pain scale for a kid who ranks major abdominal surgery as a four. So he was having a little bit of morphine. X-rays showed nothing. Scans to follow, no doubt. We're hopeful that it is a torn muscle from excessive road hockey but not dumb enough to believe our hopes. He is doing much better today (his time — same day my time). Pain flared up off the morphine, but only reached a six on the scale. It seems to be closely associated with eating. The doctors are scratching their heads and are keeping him overnight again. Then again, I think I heard that story about Will, oh, about four weeks ago.

The weird thing was hanging out at Children's with Spencer and Tracey, I had a wonderful sense of how nice it was to be home. It was short lived though. I had to run and pick up Foster from Jack and Donna's, feed him dinner, and go to a baseball meeting and pick up uniforms. I didn't find Foster, but fortunately Jack and Donna found me as I was listening to the voicemails trying to figure out where he was.

We wolfed down pizza, met the with all Foster's buddies on the team, picked up the schedule and new uniforms and then went out shopping for a new baseball glove at Canadian Tire. We picked up a bat too. Then it was practicing for spelling test, jammies, brush the teeth, pack the lunch, play a few games on the Game Cube and off to bed. Don't tell his teacher, but we skipped the fifteen minutes of mandatory reading tonight.

I guess it's like twenty-eight hours since I got out of bed this morning. Just a normal day in our strange, abnormal lives. I'm ready to call this one complete, just as soon as I phone those nice airline folks about my luggage.

Surrealia

Surrealia is a special place. As near as I can tell, it is hard place to find. To get there, you need jet lag, three quarters of a bottle of Chardonnay, Dean Martin at moderate to loud volume, and a start to the morning waking up in a hospital. But those aren't the only things. You need to be emotionally prepared as well.

Let's back up a bit. First the Spencer man. At the moment, on the scale he rates his pain as diddly-squat, which is to say he is off morphine and has been released from the hospital. As for the cause? Absolutely no frickin' idea. The important thing is that we have an entire medical team completely dedicated to making sure we go to Mexico in ten days. Right to the point of doctors and nurses willing to make the ultimate sacrifice of thirteen days at a resort on the Mayan Riviera. We have everything completely under control.

Then there is Will. I went to see him yesterday. They have me listed as immediate family, his brother. Nobody in an intensive care unit questions why a black man's brother is white or has a different last name. Will was not doing so well. Breathing on a ventilator, he had to scrawl things on a tablet. His first note started off something about Spencer. I tried to assure him that Spencer was doing okay. He became quite frantic. I was missing the point. It was a question. "Has Spencer ever been on a respirator in the ICU?" I let him know that Spencer had never been on a respirator. He seemed visibly relieved. The next scrawl was,

"Finally, I have beaten Spencer at something." So his body might be struggling, but his mind and his sense of humor remain intact.

I guess it's some kind of bond between cancer buddies. I know when Will's cancer came back and was detected a week or two ago, Spencer remarked, "That sucks, but I've done this three times now. It's no big deal."

Foster's reaction was a little different. "You never told me Will had cancer." He had absolutely no recollection of Will ever being bald from chemotherapy.

The whole thing is rather disturbing. The problem with intensive care units is that they only seem to use them for folks who need intensive care. I explained to the nurse that I was Will's brother. She said she saw the resemblance, but I know she was thinking I was a bit too old.

Anyway, Spencer is still claiming that his pain is diddly-squat. Mexico remains a possibility. A bottle of Shiraz is rapidly disappearing and I am ripping ABBA's Gold album on my way deep into Surrealia.

Scupper? Not faring so well. He started eating my staircase when he was left alone overnight. But tonight he is out walking with his buddy Boston (and Sarah and Tracey). Hopefully, he'll come around and save his neurosis until we leave him with some poor unsuspecting friends when we go to Mexico.

Gotta run. "Volare" is wrapping up and I need to let spin with "Dancing Queen".

Back to Reality

It was one of those unbelievable vacations. Entirely about fun, friends, and family. It seemed we were always busy doing something: snorkeling, swimming, jumping off cliffs at the cenotes, catching huge barracudas, swimming underground cave rivers, sailing, or scuba diving in the pool. There were long moments of contemplation lying in the shade at the beach taking long cold pulls on the straw out of my fifty-two ounce Bubba Keg, Señor Bubba as he came to be known, and contemplating really important questions like, "Why is the beach sand of an entirely uniform particle size devoid of fine silt and coarse gravel?" Enough to make you want to have another sip from Señor Bubba.

Spencer's buddy Jared was there with his family. The boys were of an age where they could tear around the resort independently and have tons of fun. Uncle John and Auntie Vicki were there with Nicole and Julia and so there were little cousins to entertain and even babysit on one evening. There were frogs and geckos to catch. Iguanas and mystery animals. Afternoon naps. Fabulous dinners.

I had a Blackberry to keep me in touch with the real world, but after a few days of checking in on complicated business and technical stuff, I decided that the real world wasn't really real and more or less ignored all the emails.

Of course vacations can't last forever. We did have to come home, which was not all bad. There was Scupper to come back to.

Foster went back to school. Spencer waved at the school and got back to his routine — chemotherapy. I returned to work.

They were nice at work. There were colleagues in town, which triggered an afternoon on Curtis' sailboat. A pleasant transition back to the work environment. I offered rides for folks after the sail and four large men climbed into Tracey's Harvest Moon Beige convertible. As we left the parking lot, I remarked to Curtis, another handsome bald man like me, "You know, this car isn't exactly a very manly car. Driving through the West End with the top down, people might get the wrong idea." He laughed.

Ten minutes later, as we were stuck in bridge traffic, there was a couple crossing the road. The husband remarked to his wife, "Oh look. They match." As he passed by the car, he began singing, "Just the Two of Us."

Yesterday, for the big meeting, I wore sandals. No socks. I brought my Bubba Keg. After all, you don't want to suffer shock from too rapid of an immersion. Nobody will ever really know whether there was Kahlua in my coffee.

Today on the way home from clinic, Spencer and Tracey stopped in to visit Will. Ten year olds aren't really supposed to be in the ICU, but I think once you've been there a couple of times yourself, you've earned the right. He wanted to go and so he did. They shared high fives. Spencer is going to get Will a bravery bead from Children's for an ambulance ride and a tracheotomy.

Maybe the real world is real after all.

Out there somewhere is a cool cenote with a cave to swim through and a white beach on the other side. It sure seemed real at the time.

The Lists

I found it a little disturbing. In our office there is a whiteboard, and on it, I found the lists. There was a "Tracey Do List" and a "Honey Do List".

There is nothing really wrong about lists in and of themselves. Let's face it, our brains are overloaded and we need some triggers for our memories, so the lists were an okay idea. I don't mind that Tracey listed things for me to do that we hadn't discussed.

I can't really complain about the amount of work. On Tracey's list there are fourteen items. On mine, only five.

I didn't feel any guilt that she has three times the number of things to do, and I don't mind that she already has eight things crossed off of her list and I've only done one. No, there is just something about the content of my list that leaves me squirming.

Here is my list:

- CDs
- Soffits
- Power wash patio
- Steve Dentist
- Vasectomy

So guess which one I've done? That's right. The patio looks good. The soffits haven't fallen down again, they just rattle a bit in a big wind. I've never even had a cavity; I don't know why I would need to go to the dentist. I guess I better put away the big pile of CDs that I ripped and then my list is substantially complete. Would it be okay to erase the whiteboard now?

Survivor Eleven — Citadel Island

First, let's start with the party. There were tribal council meetings with torches. There was the North Island and the South Island where our back yard and front yard used to be. There was the Blue Tiger Tribe and the Flames Tribe with seven boys each.

Shelters were built, points awarded. Only seven of ten lizards were recovered as the tribes scoured the neighborhood following the riddles and compass directions on the scavenger hunt. Valuable life skills were learned as marbles launched from slingshots shattered ceramic tiles. More points, more tribal council meetings, and some kind of strange dress-up relay ritual in which ten and eleven year old boys donned rubber boots, hats, shirts and bras. They learned how to take them off quickly. More valuable life skills.

Finally, there was some strange final challenge with toilet plungers. The last torch was extinguished and one team was awarded the Tiki Tiki idol.

Strangely, the most popular part of the whole party seemed to come after the cake and the gifts where the uncut tape was rolled for all to see the episode. Parents came to pick up their tribe members and all stayed to watch to the end.

Though nobody was voted off the island, I must say that Scupper better pray for immunity going into the next tribal council meeting. I'll be looking to have his torch snuffed.

Perhaps I should back up a bit. Today, Spencer was not well. Chills and mild fever. Tracey took him to the lab for blood work, and while they were out, a loaf of bread snuck out of the basket on the counter and found its way into Scupper's belly. I was called home, as Spencer and Tracey made preparations to go to Children's when the fever went over the 38.5 mark. I picked Foster and his buddy Zach up from daycare, fed them and we went to Foster's ball game. Two at bats, two hits, one run and one RBI. Good fun.

But Scupper? Not good fun. I wasn't in the mood to take him with us to the ballpark, and out of good luck or sheer brilliance on my part, I locked him in his crate. When we came home, the smell was overpowering. Scupper was designed to eat dog food, and anything else is a gastrointestinal nightmare. So it was.

I took him outside, hosed him off and gave him a good rub down with the towel. Though it wasn't pleasant, I was quite smug as I pressure washed his crate, thinking about how bad it might have been if I had left him with free range inside the house. I'm sure it wasn't pleasant for Scupper either. Losing control in your crate is totally uncool in the dog world, and when he poops he likes to have the nice squishy texture of the grass as he stomps his back feet on the ground working his way around in a big arc. Perhaps too much detail.

Meanwhile at Children's, Spencer was having a bad reaction to some IV antibiotics. His night hasn't been the peak of pleasantness. Benadryl was ordered.

As I came back in the house, I was a little disturbed that the smell was undiminished. It was a little strange. I quickly became yet more disturbed. No sign of Scupper. He wasn't guarding over

Foster in the bathroom while he showered. Then it hit me that perhaps Scupper was suffering more distress.

I called him. He didn't come. Where could he be? Perhaps in the living room, one of the few places in the house where you might find that lovely squishy texture that feels so good under your feet when all is not well in your gut.

The great circular arc of indescribable splatter told that tale. That and Scupper cowering in the corner. A full roll of paper towels, several buckets of hot soapy water, six doggy towels, and some deft work with the Shop-Vac put things in order.

Meanwhile, back at Children's, the Tylenol and antibiotics weren't breaking the fever. Tracey and Spencer were getting ready to settle in there for the night. I had bread-less sandwiches to make for lunch, a Shop Vac to empty, and of course the big decision to make: Where will Scupper sleep tonight?

Ah, I'm even willing to grant the beast immunity, as long as I can have my tribe back together to light the torches.

Beware the White Bun

The string is tied to a pop can. From there, two more pop cans are tied on. The weight of the first will drag the second two off the kitchen counter. Once three pop cans are in motion, kinetic energy is your friend. From there it escalates. Next on the string is the drain plug from the kitchen sink followed by a stainless steel beater. Not a lightweight one, but the heavy Kitchen Aid kind. It tows along its friend, which is a sixteen-ounce stainless steel travel mug. When all of that is in motion with gravity pulling down the cascade, you have enough energy for something really significant. It's a lot like a nuclear bomb. I can't just light a match; I have to direct some serious energy at the core.

The core is my friend: the fifty-two-ounce Bubba Keg. The ultimate payload.

Of course, we also need a trigger. That's where the fluffy white bun from Cobb's bread comes in. Just barely overlapping the edge of the counter, the bun is tied to the first pop can that starts the chain reaction. This is no recreational weapon system. It's a serious deterrent. This weapon system is directed at an enemy.

I was away in Dallas the first half of this week. While I was gone, I heard some disturbing telephone reports. Foremost of which was that Spencer was experiencing leg pains. So much so that he was rolling in and out of clinic for chemo on a wheelchair rather than walking. The only wheels he was using before I left were on his bike.

The other news was that Scupper was doing a little self-service lifting the lid off a pizza box and extracting a slice for personal gain. Now, there are really smart people looking after the leg pains and mild fevers. It was up to us to fix this problem, so we closed the kitchen doors, locking the enemy out of the battlefield and rigged up the apparatus described. Spencer lined up the video camera. We performed a test operation and armed the system. Then we opened the kitchen doors and headed upstairs to tuck the boys into bed with the video running. We put a gate across the stairs so Scupper couldn't follow. We all waited for the crash while we were reading stories. Hell was poised to rain down on Scupper's head.

But there was no crash, just sleepy boys. Later, Tracey reviewed the videotape. There was one shot of him raising his nose up to sniff the bun and then somehow he walked away. "He's a smart dog," Tracey told me, "I think he may be smarter than you." For a moment, I felt a sense of pride in my clever dog. Unfortunately, it wasn't until after Tracey left the room that I worked through the other interpretation of her comment. She might be right.

Then at two o'clock in the morning, as I slept soundly, Tracey heard a great crash in the kitchen. Next, the sound of little feet running back upstairs. She found Scupper on Spencer's bed trying to look sleepy as though he had no idea what the noise could be.

Today at the clinic, more chemo and more wheelchairs. Mild fevers and general malaise. They didn't let Spencer come home tonight. I'm sure Scupper would be willing to keep his bed warm. Chemo finishes tomorrow.

I Have Become Comfortably Numb

I used to be a big Pink Floyd fan. I mean, they weren't Led Zeppelin, but they were a good band. Then somehow trending towards middle age, the world became Sarah McLachlan and Diana Krall with some residual Mark Knopfler. Less Sultans of Swing and more Sailing to Philadelphia.

But not tonight. To and from my in-laws' place to install the new toilet, it was *The Wall* and *Dark Side of the Moon* as loud as the little stereo in Tracey's Harvest Moon Beige VW could crank it. Practically spiritual.

There is nothing quite like fitting a tank and pressing a new wax ring onto a pristine bowl to cleanse the mind of scan day, and nothing like pulling the old bowl and scraping the old wax ring to remind you that there is a lot of shit in life. Such was the day.

I was supposed to be in Russia today, but I didn't go. As Spencer was hobbling around last week and they scheduled a bone scan, I decided to stay home. A good man went to Russia without me and did good things, and Spencer watched *Men in Black II* as I played Spider Solitaire on my laptop. Tracey comforted a friend up on 3B who is having a day and a week and a month as bad as anything you can imagine. In relative terms, I was having a picnic in the park as cameras drifted over top of Spencer, highlighting those suspicious bits in pelvis and spine where ugly things are clearly visible and the only question is, "Are they much worse than they were last December?"

I thought I knew the answer last week without needing a scan, and then the pain went away, the bicycle came out and Spencer was back in school. We've been encouraging Spencer to pursue a new activity since it's tough to maintain a regular schedule in team sports. The dialogue took weeks, but went something like this:

"Tae Kwon Do?"

"No!"

"Guitar lessons?"

"No."

Tracey suggested bass guitar because girls really seem to go for bass players.

"Okay."

Spencer Went to Camp

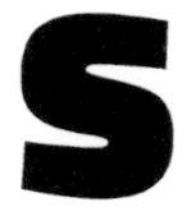pencer went to school camp.

Spencer had fun. Spencer felt not well.

Tracey went to camp.

Spencer and Tracey came home from camp and slept at home.

Spencer and Tracey and Scupper went back to camp the next day.

Fifty-two kids threw a tennis ball all day long. Scupper ran after it.

Over and over again.

Foster and Steve went to camp for family campfire night.

Steve bumped Scupper with his elbow. Scupper fell over and didn't get up again.

Foster and Steve and Scupper came home. Tracey and Spencer stayed over.

Scupper slept and slept and threw up a bunch of grass and slept again.

Spencer had fun.

Tracey and Spencer came home.

Camp was a richly rewarding experience. I think. But I wasn't really there except for the campfire, but not really because capture the flag didn't end until really late so Foster and I had to go home before the campfire. Except that there wasn't room in Lonnie's car for Scupper, so I came home with Jack and Donna and Lance and Scupper. Foster ended up staying for the campfire, and coming home later with Lonnie. Which was kind of weird, because why did I come home earlier with no kid to tuck in?

Camp was confusing.

It wasn't like that when I was a kid.

When I was a kid, I didn't go to camp, because camp was for the seventh graders. Then we moved and camp was for the sixth graders at the new school and I was grade seven, so I never got to go. Imagine if we had moved the other way. I could have gone twice. But I did go to Girl Guide camp, even though I was a boy. But that's another story. I turned out okay, and I know how to cook sausages on a twig stove made from a coffee can, which is rather a useless skill since coffee doesn't come in cans much anymore. Mostly you just buy it at Starbucks and pay four bucks for it and they don't call it coffee anymore.

The doctor called today, and Spencer's bone scan turned out okay. His disease is stable since last December, which is good news, but I wasn't worried. You can tell when I am worried because I don't write coherently.

On Strength and Courage

We met Will and Sarah because their puppy Boston is a Portuguese Water Dog and it's always polite to say hello to the humans. Now the humans are dear friends, like an aunt and uncle to the boys.

On March 3rd, Will didn't show up for my birthday party. On March 4th, he cancelled our squash game and I drove him home from the ER. By March 5th, he was back in the hospital. And for the last fifteen weeks he's been there. Mostly he has been in the ICU. His meals come in an IV bag and a machine does his breathing for him through a tracheotomy tube.

Tonight, his wife Sarah called. It was an eventful day. We had a long chat. I went back outside to share the news with Spencer as he glued together the timber twig structure for the scaled down version of the Iroquois long house.

"I talked to Sarah. They took Will to VGH today and he went to see a specialist for Myasthenia Gravis. They did a bunch of tests and they think they have figured out what is wrong with him," I said.

"Oh. What's wrong with him?" Spencer asked.

"Well, it's not Myasthenia Gravis. They think it's something else: either myositus, or polymyositus, or dermatomyositus or somethingorother. They're going to do a muscle biopsy to be sure exactly what. But it's quite rare and it's caused by his thymoma, and it's quite curable."

“Oh. Well, that’s good. What’s his thymoma?” Spencer asked.

When I was eleven, I think people were sick, and if they were really sick they were in the hospital, but that was about all I knew. Spencer is a little more medically sophisticated than your average kid.

“Thymoma is his cancer. Will is a little bit freaked about having more chemotherapy.”

“Why?”

A good question. I stood there kind of silent. Spencer has had more chemotherapy than anyone I know of. Why indeed would anybody be freaked out about chemotherapy? This is a kid who went to visit a friend on 3B last week knowing it might be his last visit. He has faced life events and treatments that make chemo seem like nothing. I didn’t have an answer for him.

“What kind of chemo?” he asked.

“Cyclophosphamide,” I explained.

“Cyclo? That’s nothing. You can’t even feel it. It’s not like they are giving him cisplatin or its ugly sister, ahh…”

“Carboplatin?” I prompted.

“Yah, carbo! It’s no big deal!”

No big deal indeed. I’d like to think that I could view the world so simply through the eyes of an eleven-year-old boy, but there is nothing simple about Spencer’s view of the world. He sees it all in ways that the rest of us can’t imagine. Instead, I would just like to have his courage. Yes, I would take Spencer’s courage or Will’s strength any day.

Go Will, Go! I’m going to book a squash court.

A Good Weekend

Right now, the suspicion is cast on me. After all, I am the only one that went anywhere near it with a sharp object. The assumption is that I am the one that did the damage. Now it doesn't work. It just hangs there and one of our primary sources of joy is gone.

Scupper's tail wags no more.

It seems permanently clamped between his legs. My guess is that I just trimmed his butt hairs a little short and he is embarrassed to wag his tail and be "naked", but it could be something worse. If it doesn't start wagging by tomorrow, it will be off to the vet. I swear I didn't do it. My guess is Tracey took Scupper for a run, then loaded him in the back of the truck and slammed the hatch on his tail. But she's not talking.

Anyway, it was a good weekend, mostly. Friday, I let the boys know that one of Spencer's friends from 3B lost his battle with cancer.

Saturday, we sent David Visschedyk off on his ride across Canada to raise money for the James Fund for neuroblastoma research. It was a small send-off on the shores of Vanier Park with a few media types. The organizers had me all prepped to talk to the TV people, but they didn't want to talk to me. After all, Spencer is eleven. He did all the talking and made the news at six and eleven. He's twice the spokesperson that I could ever be.

Then it was back home for Canada Day celebrations. Spencer and Foster set up an impromptu lemonade stand to exploit the crowds on the way to the park. It seems they mostly bussed people there this year and street traffic was down. I think the boys raised about $20 for the "oncology department at Children's Hospital" before they lost interest. They owe me $2 for lemonade mix, $5 for party ice, $4.50 for gas, and $3 to rent the patch of lawn. Once they pay that, they will understand what "proceeds" really are.

Then it was the big night of fireworks in the park, followed by a sleepover with friends in a tent, followed by an interesting educational experience in which a loud party across the street got out of hand and a girl who was rather upset about her bottle-throwing boyfriend being arrested and her own handcuffs being a little tight, used many colorful phrases that the boys had never heard before to describe exactly what she thought of the police officers. We moved the sleepover inside.

Foster lost the second of his two front teeth, so he has regained facial symmetry, but is utterly lost when it comes to corn on the cob. If the tooth fairy can ever find out where he is sleeping, I'm sure the toonie will catch up with him.

Yesterday, I went to visit Will, but he wasn't up to visitors. In the afternoon, we had a lovely time swimming and barbecuing at Uncle Vicki's and Auntie John's. Somewhere over the course of the weekend, I rode my bike about 75 km in a few laps around the Poco trail. Scupper, if I had a tail, I would be right there with you buddy.

So it was a good weekend, or at least that's the lie we tell ourselves. We tell it so often, we can't tell when we are lying. That's how we keep living. Our thoughts are with you Jesstin, and your family. Keep up the good humor, wherever you are, and forgive us for not pausing to reflect. We'll do that one day. One day when we are not terribly afraid that we won't be able to get going again after the pause.

The Mac

When your firm's best business partner calls, you do what they ask. If it means that you have to be away from your family, you do it. Sacrifice the weekend? Absolutely. Travel 1600 miles to get there? Of course. It's all about working towards mutual success and doing what is right for the relationship. Such is my level of commitment to my company and our partner.

Would I take it a step further? Without question. Drive a boat with a long metallic stick into a storm with lightning all around? The only question is, "What heading?" And as the wind clocked around seven hundred and twenty degrees and the rain came down so hard that I had to shut my eyes and steer the boat by feel alone, did I wonder what I was doing there? Not for a moment.

I am a company man.

After all, we had jumper cables running from the shrouds to the water so there was a good chance that a lightning strike wouldn't blow holes through the hull. Two and half inches of rain in twenty minutes and I think most of it went straight down my neck and into my underwear. Happy to make the sacrifice. Didn't flinch as a boat ten feet longer rounded up in front of us and was knocked flat as we surfed waves in thirty-knot winds. Just doing what had to be done. A couple of days on a few hours sleep. And proudly, I donated small portions of my liver to the cause – mostly Heineken with a touch of Mount Gay rum.

Some would call it the "Mac" – a 333-mile race up Lake Michigan. For me, it was just another business meeting.

That's my story and I'm sticking to it. Please don't tell my boss anything different. Of course, the good crew of *Outrageous* know the real truth, but they are all sworn to secrecy. They will never tell how much fun it is or how much it reminds you that you are really alive. They can never explain what it means to sail in a perfect wind under spinnaker at ten knots on a moonless night with countless meteors. Their story among other sailors will be a little different from mine. They will mention things about sailing into a big windless hole in the middle of the lake or missing the breeze on the Michigan shore and not finishing where they wanted to. But they're sailors, every one. And damn good people.

There to win? Of course. But mostly to live life as it should be lived. And so it was.

Big Projects

Our furnace never started working this fall. I did my manly things and removed the panels on the front, checked the pilot light, and changed the batteries on the thermostat. For extra effect, I pulled out my multimeter, put it on the continuity check setting, and made some impressive beeping noises. It was all show. I don't understand furnaces. I'm really hoping that with global warming we won't need one, or maybe I can find a furnace guy named Mario.

The garage door needed repair last week — a frayed cable. I do understand garage doors. It's one of the few do-it-yourself jobs where you have a chance of killing yourself. We now have two new cables, a new set of rollers, and as an extra bonus, they serviced the opener for half price. I just wanted one cable done. Three hundred and forty-seven dollars and fifteen cents. There is no name on the invoice, but I am pretty sure the guy wasn't named Mario.

As for Mario, he finished the stonework on the bottom of our chimney. It's a beautiful job. I don't even know Mario's last name or his company name. I have no written contract, have yet to see an invoice, and haven't even paid a dime for deposit. I have absolute confidence that we won't go a dime over the quote. It's just one of those trust things.

As for Spencer, he finished his PET scan, CT scan, and bone scan. Things have not improved. They are moving in the other direction. This week we follow up with a bone marrow biopsy and

MIBG scans. I haven't seen the quote yet, but it always seems to be no charge — at least in ordinary units of currency. But still we have to go back and back for rework. It's definitely not a do-it-yourself job, but it's otherwise a lot like garage doors.

Spencer thinks it may be a do-it-yourself job, or at least it has a heavy do-it-yourself component.

Foster was struggling with his homework the other night. "I can't do it. I can't do it!"

Spencer jumped in, "Yes you can. You can do anything you want. If you say you can't, you won't. But if you think you can, you'll be amazed at what you can do."

Foster thought about it for a while. "How come you haven't cured your cancer then?"

"It's not like that, Foster," Spencer replied. "It's a big project and it takes a long time."

We've never met an oncologist named Mario. I think Spencer might have the right idea.

From Russia with Love

I missed Halloween. In Yaroslavl, they don't celebrate it. I never know when is a good time to travel so sometimes all I can do is make my best guess that things will be okay at home and go.

Monday night, Tuesday morning where I was, I received a disturbing email. Tracey meant to send it to Spencer's teachers, but missed by one entry on the address list and it came to me: "Serge and Stephanie, Spencer had to start his chemo treatment today as he started experiencing quite severe pains in his legs and back last night. He asked to go to the hospital this morning and they have been able to manage his pain with morphine. Hopefully, the chemo will start doing its job soon and the pain meds won't be needed. He won't be at school tomorrow or the rest of the week. Tracey."

This wasn't the way the week was supposed to turn out, but you make the best of it. For Spencer, that meant a call to his photographer. John from the *Globe and Mail* is doing a photo essay on Spencer as part of a huge national feature on cancer. The plan for the day was for photos at the school in Halloween costume, but instead it was photos in the clinic with IV pole. Either way is part of the real daily life of a kid with cancer.

By Tuesday afternoon, Spencer was ready for trick or treating. They cheated a little bit and Spencer had some Tylenol to knock down a fever so he could leave the clinic rather than being admitted for IV antibiotics. Then it was off home where good neighbors had delivered and carved a 300-pound pumpkin. Onward to terrorize the neighborhood in full pirate regalia demanding candy.

Meanwhile, back in Yaroslavl, I did what I do best. That is, I pretended everything is okay and pressed ahead. I had business meetings, and they went well. Very well. Maybe as good as business meetings ever go. We went out for dinner and celebration, and we drank vodka and toasted Canada's victory over the Soviet Union in the 1972 series. We toasted Russia's victories over Canada in other years, which I claim not to remember. We went out and played billiards, a familiar game of eight ball and a Russian game on a larger table with all white balls and narrow pockets. After a final toast for the evening, I said goodbye to Sergei, Alexey, Roman, and Maxim, and I was alone at my hotel.

The world was spinning a little bit, so I went out for a walk in the cold night air to clear my head. A police car came around the corner and stopped as I crossed the street behind it. I heard words behind me in Russian that I did not understand so I kept walking.

This was a mistake.

Soon I heard very loud words behind me and I turned to see the police coming toward me with their guns. I thought it would be good to show them some identification since I could not communicate with them and went to reach for my passport.

This was a bigger mistake.

Now I had a pistol pointed at my head and automatic rifle poking my ribs and the language was very loud. I turned around and put my hands on the railing.

This was the right thing to do.

They searched me and found my wallet and spent a fair amount of time looking through it, yelling at me any time I turned around to make sure they weren't stealing my cash. They asked me many questions, none of which I understood. After five or ten minutes, there was one question that I did get, "Canada?"

"Yes, I am from Canada," I said. They asked some other question and pointed at the hotel. "Yes, I am staying at the hotel," I said. The language became quieter and they got back in their car.

Apparently, my haircut is a little unusual in Russia. It is more in the style of the once popular Russian mafia, so as I wander the streets alone in the early hours of the morning, I look a little more like a dangerous threat to society than a visiting foreign businessman. Next time, I will wear a hat.

Spencer finished off Halloween by checking into Children's. I finished off two more days of meetings in Moscow and said goodbye to some great people and a great country and took an early flight home.

Only twenty-seven hours after leaving my hotel, I am here in a cot next to Spencer on the ward in 3B. It is good to be home, but a little disturbing. Armed men point automatic weapons and shout at me in Russian and it doesn't even rate at the top of the list of scary things for the week.

Sucking the Fun Out

Somehow we got it in our minds that we might have to vacate our house if the restoration people had to open up walls and there was any chance that Spencer might get exposed to mould. Being forced out of your family home and into a hotel is not a terribly good feeling.

We don't like being victims.

Now, if you leave the country and stay at a hotel next to Disneyland, you're in control of your life and not a victim, right? That was our thinking. Soon, the focus was all about Disneyland and when would be the best timing between chemo rounds. One thing lead to another and schedules were guided more by child life experts and oncologists than restoration contractors. We found ourselves on a plane to California.

For Spencer, Foster, and Tracey, the whole thing was pure fun. For me, amusement park rides are pure terror. I survived the first day. With encouragement from Spencer and Foster, I braved Space Mountain, Big Thunder Railroad, and any other ride in Disneyland that had a long line up in front of it that we could bypass with Spencer's Guest Assistance Pass. Unfortunately, the big Swiss mountain thingy was closed for seasonal repairs. What a shame.

It was day two that held the potential for real terror. That was California Adventure. Day two was the Tower of Terror and California Screamin'. I thought the Tower of Terror was a haunted house, so I willingly walked into it. I had no idea. California

Screamin' is billed as a high-speed roller coaster. It has a damn loop and you go upside down. They tried to persuade me to go on. Tracey whispered something in Spencer's ear. Soon I heard the words, "Dad, if you really love me, you'll come on this ride."

The shoulder restraints kept me from jumping out. My screams weren't loud enough to get them to stop the car as we rolled out of the loading area.

The only problem with California Screamin' was the pictures. Spencer was in the back seat and we couldn't see his face, so we went again. Tracey had her eyes closed in the next run, so we went again. Soon I was immune. Finally, we got the good picture, but they couldn't get me to go on Maliboomer. It was strictly a matter of policy. I don't do rides with built in barf shields. Tracey, Spencer and Foster went at least three times.

We tried to fly home on Monday, but there was a small weather problem in Vancouver. The precipitation was frozen into flakes. No planes were landing. But yesterday we made it. Spencer and Tracey rode in a fellow traveller's limousine straight to Children's Hospital. Chemo was overdue. Jack drove me and Foster home, squealing all the way at the prospect of six inches of untouched snow in the yard. Foster, not me or Jack. Good people had shoveled our driveway, and others looked after Scupper, even claiming that he hadn't eaten anything he wasn't supposed to. Everybody looked after us.

The restoration people had completed six days of work at our house. They had placed exactly two pieces of green tape on a piece of crown molding to flag it for removal. Everybody had a great time and it was a perfect break from the rain and the hospital and dehumidifying extraction fans. I have no idea how the boys came up with the expression, "Oh Dad, that fart could suck all the fun out of Disneyland!"

It's My Life

If you don't know me well, you might think that I don't have a good life. My name is Spencer Dolling. When I was six years old, I was diagnosed with cancer. The cancer is called stage 4 neuroblastoma. It is a solid tumor cancer that usually spreads to bones. It is rare. In BC, 130 kids are diagnosed with cancer each year. Only five kids will have stage 4 neuroblastoma. Because it isn't too common, not much research money goes to finding better medicines for this type of cancer.

Right now, most people don't think that my life is very good. If you were me, you would think otherwise. My life is great because I have three of the best friends in the world. My friends are Jared, Keaton and Michael and I've known them almost all of my life. My friends are the best because they don't care whether I'm sick or not. They will come play hockey, video games or just chat. I go to school with Jared and Keaton at Pitt River Middle School in early French immersion. My family is also the best. I have my dad Steve, my mom Tracey, my brother Foster and Scupper my dog that is hyper. My family is the best because they all love me. Foster will never admit it, same with Scupper, except he can't talk he just barks and woofs.

I started learning bass guitar this year. Sometimes I play bass guitar with Michael. Michael plays the electric guitar and we have the same teacher. Our teacher teaches us the music we like. Michael and I like the same music. One of my favorite groups is All American Rejects.

I have met a lot of the Vancouver Canucks. Trevor Linden and Dan Cloutier sang "Happy Birthday" to me on my ninth birthday. They aren't the best singers, but they are great hockey players. Sometimes I get hockey tickets from the hospital. One day I want to meet Roberto Luongo.

My family has a sailboat. During the summer, we go sailing. It is very fun. When we go on our boat, we fish, swim and beach comb. Sometimes my dad lets us go out on the dingy to cruise around sailing or motoring. Sometimes we meet up with my friend Hadley on their boat.

I have an electric go-kart, which is very fun. When I was first diagnosed, my uncles John, John, and Ron (also known as the "Ohns"), built the go-kart for me and my brother. It has a cannon that shoots tennis balls. Scupper, my dog, loves to fetch balls that shoot out of the cannon. Sometimes they shoot too far, and then Scupper can't find them. Then we send Foster running down the hill to help Scupper. Sometimes, Foster, Scupper and I have races to see who can find the ball first. At one time, we had water on the go-kart so we could shoot a water rocket or give the dog a drink.

At the hospital, I have lots of treatments. I have chemotherapy, blood transfusion, and lots of tests and scans of my body. There are great doctors, nurses and child-life specialists at the hospital. The funniest thing that happened at the hospital was when my nurse Allan blew up a glove over his head, had medicine cups sitting on his eye sockets and was acting like a chicken.

Apart from my cancer, you can see that I have a fantastic life.

(Spencer Dolling, Age 11, as printed in the *Globe and Mail*)

Reveille

Will, outstanding send-off!

Wow. All I can say is that I want to join the RCMP before I die. What Ray did on the saxophone and what Mikey and Sarah did with music and slides: unbelievable. But the eulogy, Will, that one almost didn't make it. I have to share the story with you because you would have appreciated it.

At 7:45 this morning, the phone rings. We're still asleep and I hear Tracey say, "Oh um, yes, one moment please," and she handed the phone to me. It was Chaplain Turner from the RCMP. Will, the police never call me at 7:45 in the morning. The clergy never call me. But to have them both unified in one voice, you can bet I was out of bed and on my feet in a moment.

He wanted to chat about the eulogy and asked me how long it was. I told him it was twenty-five minutes — I read it to the boys last night and Foster timed it. In Chaplain Turner's experience, twenty-five minutes turns into thirty-five by the time you factor in the emotion, and soon you've lost the group and driven ceremonies over an hour. Did I have a copy handy to discuss some edits for consideration?

Will, I'm buck-naked standing in the dark in my bedroom. "Why yes, of course, just a moment." I grabbed what I thought was underwear and ran downstairs and in no time I'm sitting in my office with your eulogy in front of me, a pair socks in my hand, talking to Chaplain Turner on the phone completely naked.

So we made a few cuts. Forgive me, Will. Satchmo and Boston didn't make it, but all of this happened before I had any coffee.

None of this put your eulogy at risk. It was the piper that undid me. I was doing great until the piper. Sarah said yes to the piper because you would have loved it. Then the piper made my tears flow, and there I sat wondering if I would ever be able to get up and speak.

But I did and I think we got it about right. I discussed targets with Ray and he was looking for about a 50/50 laughter-tears ratio and think we nailed it. I've never had a hundred guys in red uniforms shake my hand before so it must have been okay. I think you would have liked it.

Hope you're well.

Fever

As I was waking up the other morning, six anxious looking women stormed into the room. Generally, this would just be some kind of fantasy dream, but in this case, it was real. Spencer's IV pump was beeping away and I was trying to retrieve his call button that was stuck underneath the head of his bed. Somehow, by yanking on the cord I had triggered some kind of code that brought every nurse on the ward into the room. They all looked at me a little funny when I went out to get a coffee a few minutes later. We were in the hospital because Spencer had some kind of infection in his leg. It was only a couple of days in the hospital. Mild fever at the start. Seems to have sorted itself out.

My own fever hasn't subsided. I sold the sailboat that has been in Tracey's family for forty years. So far, the family doesn't hate me for it. I keep showing them pictures of a Catalina 34 that seems to keep the knives in the drawer. The nice thing about having a forty-year-old boat is that you can look at a twenty-year-old boat and it seems brand new. We have an offer on one now.

Tracey left the boys and me. I'm now doing the single parent thing for a full week. She went to Mexico with Sarah. Both of them deserve a break! About now, they should be somewhere south of Cancun having their first drink of something with an umbrella in it.

We miss her already. We've tried to numb our loss at Costco and Home Depot. We threw out all the rusty old tools in the boat toolbox and replaced them with shiny new ones. We just had pizza for dinner. Now we'll watch a hockey game. It's going to be a brutal week, but we boys will do our best.

Questions

So while Tracey and Sarah are unwinding and grieving in Mexico, a few questions have arisen that are probably better not asked of Tracey while she enjoys the beach:

- We've run out of liquid dish soap. Should we just stack pots in the sink or should we only be microwaving food in bowls that we eat out of?
- We're running out of dishwasher soap. This could be really bad. Where are the paper plates stored?
- When Foster came out of the bathroom announcing that he had thrown up, I made him put his clothes in the laundry and take a shower. Was there anything else I should have done?
- I'm trying to serve balanced meals. Tater Tots are a vegetable, right?
- The dog seems to be mining for empty toilet paper rolls in the bathroom wastebasket. I forget what this signifies. Is he lonely, bored, or underfed?
- As we arrived at the orthodontist today, my cell phone rang and I ended up talking to a customer for twenty minutes. Jared, Foster and Spencer went in, did the appointment, and came out again. What happens at the orthodontist? Was I supposed to do anything in there?

- Do the teachers consider hockey games homework? Even if they're Eastern Conference games? What if Foster is now able to spell Tampa Bay Lightning?
- How do I explain to the children the bra that was thrown on the ice after Cowan's second goal?
- Hypothetically speaking, not that this would ever happen, but if Spencer were to miss one of his antibiotic pills at dinner, would we just give him two at bedtime, throw one in the garbage and never mention it, or just carry on the usual schedule being diligent not to miss another one?

Mongolian Razor Back

Scupper didn't do so well at Balding for Dollars.

For Spencer, there was no detectable change – no need to even bother with the trimmers. He's fully committed to the cause, full time.

For Foster, well, he has a good looking head and often has short hair this time of year anyway. Looks pretty good bald.

For me, well, I always have a clean-shaven head. I tried to grow it back for a few weeks just so I'd have something to shave, but every year there is less of it and there doesn't seem to be much color left in what does come back.

Tracey is strictly off limits. She would shave her head, but we like her the way she is.

If we were going to raise any money, that pretty much left Scupper. Yep. He was our only chance to do something dramatic that would attract some attention.

The question was what to do? Bald dogs are kind of creepy. We decided not to make him look like a sick puppy. We went with a more stylized approach. We decided on a Mohawk. For the event at Children's, I just did his head and left a big bit down the middle.

There was a problem with it though. With the big shaggy ears he kind of looked like a freaky 1970s rocker, sort of dog version of Gene Simmons. I couldn't bear to look at him.

I had to finish the job, so off came the ears. I took the Mohawk all the way back to the tail. Now he really looks like something. We're not sure what exactly — part dinosaur, part mutant poodle. I want to join the Portuguese Water Dog Club, just to see the looks of shock and horror. At least now I don't have to explain all the stuff about water dogs to people we bump into on the sidewalk. It's much simpler now. I just look them in the eye and explain: "He's a Mongolian Razor Back. Don't get too close!"

Strep Yoga

I'm very excited. Tomorrow night is candle light yoga. Tracey is convinced of how good yoga would be for me. She sees candle light night as the perfect opportunity to introduce me to the art form. I think that she hopes I will enjoy it as much she does. I think she is delusional. The only reason I would go is because I love her. The only reason I would stay would be a group of women in yoga tights. We'll see how it goes.

Spencer had his birthday on the twelfth. I can't believe he is twelve already. Instead of a birthday party this year, he got to take a few friends for an overnight cruise on the boat. It seemed to be a hit. Only one fish died, and no crabs were harmed. The pirate flag was raised, but no pirates found my rum supply. No harm came to the Mongolian Razor Back.

Strep throat is everything that they say it is. I tried it out this week. If I were smart, I would have gone to my doctor early to get antibiotics that act right away and get rid of the symptoms. But I'm not, so I waited and about all the antibiotics do is make you no longer contagious. I get to experience how high my pain threshold is.

I was starting to get better but couldn't sleep at night, so the other night Tracey gave me some magic pill that pretty much knocked me out for ten hours. That was great for the drowsiness thing, but when I woke up after snoring for ten hours with strep throat, I felt like I would rather be in a yoga class. Maybe even a candle-light yoga class.

Spencer had chemo last week. I think chemo and yoga have a lot in common, but I've done neither, so I shouldn't judge. I did, however, get to go to the lab this week with Spencer. We had father son blood work. I persuaded him to go with the Donald Duck Band-Aid so he could look like me.

Foster has been playing a lot of baseball. His team is undefeated. He's thinking maybe they will win every game this year. I told him I thought that was kind of sad because he wouldn't really learn much if all they ever do is win. He's says he is quite happy not learning anything if it means they get to win every game. I wonder if I will win at yoga?

Yoga Follow Up

And I was so looking forward to it.

Unfortunately, Tracey had a little headache that she thought might develop into a migraine on Friday night. This meant that we were unable to go to candlelight yoga. It's a shame because I think there was, like, this cosmic window that opened that would have allowed me to go if it happened on Friday. I can think of no point in the past or future where the window might open again and I might be persuaded to do candlelight yoga. So I guess we're done with that topic.

Friday, I brought home a new chartplotter. It's a little screen that listens to satellites and puts a picture of your boat on a little electronic map. Vitally important for safety to know where you are. Plus, it also happens to have a fishfinder, pardon me, a depth-finding sonar that can point out how much water you have under your boat so it doesn't meet the land. Again, vitally important for safety.

So the question came. "How much did it cost?"

These questions are best never answered directly. No good can come of it. "It was on sale," I answered.

I'm glad Garmin has this figured out already. They publish a price that is designed solely for the purpose of showing your spouse. It has nothing to do with what the real cost is. You have to add in the little chip that has electronic map on it, and of course you need to add on the cost of the depth transducer. Then the lowest cost one has such a ridiculously small screen that it really makes sense to go the next size larger, also on sale of course. But since I'd already dodged the question, none of this would be exposed.

I hadn't really dodged it. The question came back again twenty minutes later. "So how much was it?" I had to explain about looking at the unit in the store and by the time you display your data, you're left looking at a chart size of a video iPod and how I didn't want to endanger our lives with such a small screen (this argument doesn't work for fifty-inch plasmas for the family room) and that I would not want to make such an investment and end up regretting it for years. The extra $200 was really worth it. What a shame that the 178c was discontinued, because now you have to buy the expensive G2 charts.

I went on and on until Tracey grew tired of the outrageous stories and I never had to answer the question.

I was showing it to Spencer, and he was suitably impressed. Then he asked, "So Dad, where's the button that you press in an emergency that makes the coast guard come?"

"Well, actually Spence, the chartplotter doesn't have a button like that. What it has is a NEMA 0183 interface that will feed the position data to a VHF radio with DSC capability that broadcasts the distress call with your position."

"You mean we would have to buy a new radio?" he asked.

This kid is smart. Scary smart. But I see the radios advertised at very reasonable prices. I'm sure they come fully accessorized with everything you need included in the price.

I've hidden the invoice, but there's no hiding the MasterCard bill. Damn. I'm going to have to go to a candlelight yoga class to make reparations.

Unbounded Perpetual Joy

Spencer wanted to get a helicopter ride. I explained that this wasn't possible.

He did, however, persuade the ambulance driver to stop at Wendy's to get chicken strips and fries. Hmmm. Perhaps I should back up a bit.

He was in the ambulance to go from Children's to the cancer clinic for radiation treatment. Since he can't walk, they arranged for an ambulance rather than Tracey having to carry him through the parking lot.

Whoops. I guess I really haven't updated in a while. He was admitted to Children's after the kayaking on Wednesday. The boys skipped out of school on Foster's birthday and went up to Sasamat Lake to have a paddle in their new inflatable kayaks that they somehow scammed out of me on Father's Day. We had dropped into West Marine to pick up some canvas snaps and these inflatable kayaks were on sale for the last day and if I would only pay half like a good father they would experience unbounded perpetual joy.

I wasn't sure we could afford to save that much money. Nonetheless, they have the kayaks and I'm still waiting to see their cash.

But the kayaks have nothing to with hospitalization. At first, I thought it was the road hockey. Monday, we had a little bit of a birthday celebration for Foster and the boys played road hockey for a couple of hours. Spencer thought he had pulled a groin muscle. Turns out it is some kind of infection in his leg. They call it cellulitis or some such fancy name. He has been on an ever-escalating course of antibiotics that have him in the hospital. No worries. A little morphine and his pain has been controlled. He is really doing okay. If you want to see him, just check out BCTV on Monday night — I think they'll run the piece at 5 and 7 pm.

Oh boy. The more I explain, the more questions there are. The radiation is targeting a bit of tumor high up in his spine. He had scans a few weeks back and things were generally improved except for this one little bit where a touch of neuroblastoma has sort of got the idea that it would like to move into his spinal cord. The doctors don't think that's such a good idea. Something about it being good to keep walking, breathing, and stuff like that. That's why they're nuking it.

The TV thing was just an interview at an EA Sports party in the lounge today. Just the local gaming studio throwing a party and spoiling kids with games and prizes and things. They're constantly doing good things for the kids, though usually not with any publicity.

Anyway, all is well and they're hopeful that Spencer won't have to have surgery next week and if he tries to walk a bit and keep the blood flowing, that's a good thing. Gotta run. We're home on a pass for a few hours. I think we'll try to play a little road hockey.

More Unbounded Perpetual Joy

The infection in Spencer's leg is not getting any smaller. It's a bit larger, but not quite so red. No fevers. The pain is much better. I think he went today without codeine and he's able to walk around with relative ease.

Since it hasn't improved to the degree that they would like with the heavy-duty antibiotics, they sent the surgery team around today to consult. The concern is that maybe the infection has gone out of the skin and into the muscle and perhaps it would be a good idea to cut away the infected tissue to help it heal. We're talking about an area the size of a DVD, so this doesn't really sound like much fun. Carving up boys never sounds like much fun.

The surgeon dropped by. She wasn't wild about the idea. Spencer didn't jump high enough when she poked it, so it's probably not a really deep nasty thing. Surgery would rather keep a close eye on it for a few days than sharpen their scalpels. You gotta like a mechanic who tells you not to worry about the noise unless it gets worse rather than pulling your wheels off, replacing your brakes, and charging you $500.

Hopefully, we'll stop drawing concentric lines soon. We did escape on a day pass for dinner again today, but it's always nice to check out for good with your boy and all his bits.

Following Seas

Sometime between being discharged from hospital last Tuesday and starting a new round of chemotherapy today, there were a few days of indescribable perfection. They involved some things like a small shark on the end of some ten pound test, wind shrieking through the rigging on an undersized anchor at 3:00 am, kayaking in a cove named Smugglers, smokies on a fire in Buccaneer Bay, racing in Secret Cove, meeting up with friends, and sailing home surfing on a following sea in a twenty knot north west. And other things.

Today there is chemotherapy and the realization that I'm falling behind on the maintenance items. The wiring needs to be fixed for the passenger window, the brakes shudder at high speed, the timing belt is overdue for replacement, I need to get a root canal, the vasectomy is still on the list, and I really must rebuild the front porch with the cedar and stone.

It all seems a little overwhelming. I should break it down into smaller pieces. I think I'll phone Mario and book the car in for service. Yep, I'll tackle the tough one first and the rest will be easy.

Maintenance

I've made good progress on the maintenance backlog. I booked the car in this week and rode the Skytrain for a couple of days. Mario did a fabulous job. He did everything I asked for at about half the price of what the dealer would charge. What I really like is that he did a couple of things that I didn't ask for. He fixed the rattly clunky noise underneath with a new sway bar linkage. Best of all, when he restored the 1, 2 & 3 settings on my air conditioner fan with a new resistor (not an expensive new assembly) as I asked, he also managed to make the thing stop squealing as an added bonus.

Now that I've got the tough one out of the way, I've started in on the next steps. I called the endodontist to book an appointment. I explained that Dr. Johnson said I needed to meet with Dr. Weinstock personally because I had a non-vital 3-2 that may be trifurcated. The receptionist was impressed. "We don't see that very often."

"I know. Arnie even dragged his associate in and said, 'you have to have a look at this'. That's never a good sign." The receptionist explained their approach to fees. They charge more than the fee guide recommends, and they like to extract cash from the patient rather than waiting for the insurance company to pay them.

What are the options here? They kind of have you by the short and curlies. Never mind, that's the other health care professional. In any case, it sounds like it will be expensive. I suppose you don't really want to go for a discount root canal. Especially when it's your first, and a complicated one.

Now I'm a little bit alarmed. I find that the less I pay for car repairs, the better quality service I get. Does the same hold true in dentistry? I don't want to find out the hard way.

The alarming bit is lower down, and I don't know why, but people are distinctly uncomfortable when I start talking about my pending vasectomy. I'm not at all uncomfortable talking about it. I'm uncomfortable with the notion of doing it. Especially when the price is zero. Discounted car repairs — for sure. A discount on a root canal — I don't know. But rendering yourself reproductively inert for free? This sounds like a bad idea. What if they tell me it's non-vital or trifurcated?

Saving Room in the Bucket

I would like to tell everyone about the wonderful vacation and all the things that we did and make people generally jealous or inspired or whatever. Not just the, "Isn't it nice that the cancer family got away for a couple of weeks?" but more along the lines of, "Oh my God, why can't we have vacations like that?"

I should natter on about the fifteen knot breeze on the flat water rounding Shark Spit with the sun low in the western sky and the sails full and the boat nicely heeled and try to express in words what it feels like when you know in your heart that you're living one of life's great moments and it doesn't get any better. And the clams in the lagoon off Manson's Landing where we dug our limit of 225 in ten minutes with our hands and didn't even disturb more than four square feet of sand. And the stunning solo anchorage in Grace Harbour where the boys managed to find the perfect rocks for us to jump from. And rock crabs with white wine. And watching the boys jump off the top deck of Al and Sue's boat with four life jackets and two boat cushions on so they hit the water like wine corks at terminal velocity. And the biscuits, the ones that went with the chowder of prawns and clams and fresh cod. Swimming in the lakes. Kayaking. The little dog named Pepper. And Foster's octopus, which stayed with us not quite long enough to be given a name before going back to the deep. And just sailing from one cove to the next with those perfect hours where Spencer devoured the new *Harry Potter*, only disturbed occasionally when there might be a cry of "Dolphins!"

But I won't. Because it would be misleading. Life isn't entirely perfect.

Sometimes it's only moments of perfection otherwise encapsulated in crap.

Because in reality we didn't even know if we were going to get away or not. The days before we left, Spencer had a fever and was in the hospital getting transfusions and IV antibiotics. On the way up, we stopped in Powell River. Foster and I went shopping while Tracey and Spencer went for blood work so we could be sure that platelets were stable enough for us to disappear into the wilds of Desolation Sound.

Ten or twelve days of perfection, and on the way back, more fevers and back pains and a stop in Nanaimo Hospital for more IV antibiotics. It would be nice if the antibiotics were fighting infection, but they were only a precaution. The cultures were negative. The pain and the fevers are the cancer, and when we got home it got worse. Much worse. Tylenol and codeine weren't cutting it. Spencer asked to be taken to hospital in agony. IV morphine did the trick.

Today, there was a bone marrow biopsy and a new plan, and the pain is better managed. New chemo is flowing. Tomorrow, Tracey is organizing a barbecue, because there are too many kids and parents on 3B stuck inside their rooms on beautiful summer days. Fear is replaced by hope and we move forward.

The real trick is to encapsulate the crap and let the enjoyment of the moments triumph. Otherwise, you're just stuck in a bucket of shit, and you really need the bucket for the rock crabs and the octopus.

Learn 'em Good

My job is to teach life's important lessons.

The other night the supply of premium toilet paper that Sarah left us when she packed up and sold her place was exhausted. Foster was wrapping things up on a number two and whined, "Hey, this isn't Charmin Ultra." I sensed a learning moment.

"Be grateful, Foster," I explained, "When I was a kid, we didn't have toilet paper. We had to get by with leftover sixty-grit from the mill down the road."

"That can't be true, Dad. Sand paper wouldn't even flush down the toilet."

"Ah, who said anything about flush toilets? When I was a kid, we had pit toilets and they were thirty-eight feet deep."

"You did not."

"Yes we did. In fact, I used to have two other brothers. They were both lost to pit toilet accidents. The only reason uncle Ron survived is because he had a big butt." None of this was true of course. It seemed like an important lesson at the time. Sometimes a learning moment can go bad.

This weekend, Spencer was reeling in a big salmon when a fisheries patrol vessel came charging by. I don't think we've seen a fisheries patrol vessel in twenty years, but when they saw Spencer's rod bent over they decided to come by for a chat. With their large wake and much confusion, we somehow lost the fish before we saw it. Such is fishing. They wanted to have a look at our licenses and our gear. In spite of a very lax enforcement environment over the years, we've maintained a semi-rigorous approach to compliance with the fisheries laws. The rod on the port side of the boat had the regulation barbless hooks. The rod on the starboard side had a somewhat older hoochie with the recently outlawed barbed hooks. These would have worked their way through inventory and disappeared in a season or two. We're content in the knowledge that we generally represent no threat to the salmon population and if the fisheries law is a few years ahead of us, we know we'll catch up to it eventually.

However, with three enthusiastic officers wanting to board our vessel, I didn't have a couple of years. Thankfully, Tracey suggested to them that she would just tack the boat into the wind so we wouldn't blow off as they tried to board. With the boom swinging and a two-foot chop, we were looking a little dangerous. I graciously put fenders out on the port side even though they came up on our starboard. They came around to the port side, decided not to board, and just hovered off five to ten feet away. I showed them licenses (all current, though the boys don't have salmon tags on theirs), and explained our gear. "Yep, we're using flashers with hoochies and look, no barbs," as I held up the newer hoochie and ran my thumb over the hook where barbs might be. I didn't volunteer to show them the other rig — a representative sample seemed sufficient.

"Oh good. You just saved yourself a hundred and fifty bucks. That's what it would cost if you were fishing with barbs." They gave us a few words about what species were running and why we shouldn't lose any fish with barbless hooks if we just keep the tension on, etc. We smiled, waved and sent them on their way. Technically, I didn't lie to the fisheries officers. I just didn't volunteer the whole truth. Another great lesson for the boys.

I dropped into the clinic today. Unfortunately, Spencer is having pain in his back again. Not nearly the right ratio of fun days to hospital days lately. More chemo to start next week. He is starting on a study for an appetite stimulant. They collected baseline data on his quality of life, took his height and weight, measured the circumference of his arm, and then the dietician tried to squeeze some fat on his arm so she could get her calipers on it. Spencer was writhing in pain. There was no fat to squeeze. She felt the need to try again. She left a nice bruise on his arm. She had to be told to stop and she left the room. We all stared in wonder at the bruise forming on his arm. The wonder only lasted a moment or two before the nurse, doctor, Tracey and I all started speculating on what his platelet number would be. It was one of those *Price is Right,* closest to the number without going over kind of moments, so I chose seven — something just north of spontaneous bleeding out of the ears.

Thankfully, we were all wrong. Spencer seems to be manufacturing his own platelets again and scored in the fifties! At lunch, Tracey mentioned that Foster was pretty bummed because he felt a little cheated out of his summer with the recent bad weather and what not. Spencer mentioned that he never had a chance to go go-kart racing again. And so was hatched a plan in which Spencer didn't go back to school that afternoon, I didn't go back to work, we dragged Foster out of class and we all went go-kart racing. Another good lesson in how to deal with adversity: just drop your responsibilities and go have some fun. What am I teaching my children?

Wilmington Tan

Spencer just finished a seven-day round of chemo. The last two days were inpatient for the vincristine / doxo Kool-Aid combo. The last go around the planned two days stretched into twenty-two days, so it was great to be free on time. I think Spencer even plans to go back to school tomorrow for a day or so until his counts bottom out.

Foster and I were charged with painting the family room while Spencer was in hospital. It didn't start out so well as I was giving a paint can a little shake when it leapt out of my hands and burst open on to the family room floor. A full gallon. It took a lot of swearing before we managed to salvage the paint from the floor and get it on the walls. On the bright side, Foster can use a roller without any lap marks and he now knows how to use the "F" word as a noun, a verb, an adverb, and an adjective. I taught him myself.

Scupper had a bath today. Tracey keeps raving about how cute he is. I'm still struggling with the relevance of cute when he had to have the patch of Benjamin Moore Wilmington Tan latex cut out of his hide at the point where he rubbed against my newly painted wall. Although I suppose cute keeps me from killing him.

Therapy

I could see him driving up the shoulder a full block behind me. He was obviously somebody whose time was much more valuable than the rest of us stuck in traffic.

I took the opportunity to drift right a bit. Okay, a lot. To the point where there was no way he could get past me. As he approached, rather than merging in, he honked at me, mistaking an ambush predator for some geriatric driver with lane keeping incontinence. I moved left a bit — just enough that he could squeeze through, but only as far as my mirror.

I lowered my passenger side window. I screamed at the top of my lungs, "You're driving in the bicycle lane, dickhead!"

It felt fantastic. Therapeutic asshole-ism. I highly recommend it.

But you have to practice carefully. A colleague dropped into my office to talk about a quality problem for one of our customers. I interrupted before he could say anything. "Hold on just a second," I said. I pulled out a roll of finely honed carving chisels that I had brought in for pumpkin carving. I unrolled them on my desk and arranged them in front of me. I selected a large gouge and carefully shaved the hair off the back of my knuckles to demonstrate the sharpness. I put the gouge down. "Okay, go ahead."

My boss explained to me that it's only fun if both the people are enjoying it. You can't practice therapeutic asshole-ism at work. I rode my bike to work the next day. I do it every now and then. It takes an hour and twenty minutes, and there is no anger left after riding that long. People probably think I have a new love for the environment, or perhaps I have some major new fitness thing going on. Maybe they think I just like to wear the stretchy pants.

If only they really understood. I am protecting them from my inner asshole. Then there's the outer one. That which soothes the inner chafes the outer (even with the cushy pad in my stretchy pants). We must all strive to keep our assholes in balance.

A New Era

We're running out of options in Canada and we are about to enter a new era. Everything is different now.

I've given my MasterCard number to an out-of-country hospital.

It doesn't leave me with a warm feeling. It's just one step above sending my bank account numbers to someone in Nigeria introduced through email offering mutual benefit.

But there is a human on the other end of the line. Wendy is the Patient Financial Specialist. We don't speak to a medical specialist; they have to process the $500 consultation fee before that happens. Wendy promises she will never process a payment on my card without discussing it with me first. I believe her. She hasn't asked me for my bank account numbers yet.

Wendy is just waiting to hear back from the doctor about an opening in her schedule this week for us to go and discuss what treatment options are available in the US. We're bringing our medical people with us: oncologist and nurse — we're going fully loaded. We'll squeeze a full day of professional development out of the $500 consultation fee.

"Okay, just let us know," I say to Wendy. "We're on a bit of a tight schedule and want to get things arranged. I've borrowed my sister's mini-van and we're ready to roll whenever you say."

"I'll let you know as soon as I hear," Wendy advises. "And I just have one more item to get costed and as soon as I have the sedation numbers, I'll have that estimate ready for you." Wendy is pricing out a big job for us. The clinical trial is free, but that's just the marketing department sucking you in. You still have to pay for all the scans and bone marrow biopsies and ancillary stuff that goes along with a month-long visit.

"Oh great. That was the other question Tracey had. Let me know the numbers when you get them. I think we'll probably just sell my sister's minivan instead of giving it back to her."

Wendy didn't even laugh. She must have thought that it was normal for people to sell their assets to pay for treatment. Yikes!

Please Send More Minivans

Dear Vicki:

Thanks for the minivan. I had hoped to get it back to you before you returned from your trip, but there was a small problem, and I had to sell it. I hope you don't mind. It was a nice minivan, what with the leather guts and everything, but it was a little long in the tooth so I could only get $15,000 for it.

Turns out the problem is a little bigger than I thought.

We've been dealing with Wendy. Nice lady. She is able to offer us not one, but up to three different clinical trials. The trials are totally free. All we need to pay for are the scans, bone marrow biopsies, bandages, gauze, etc. You see, none of the Canadian scans, biopsies, etc., are any good because well, they're free, and how could they possibly be any good? Depending on which trial we're on, they will offer everything for the low cost of $76,000 to $86,000 US. And it includes the use of the outpatient bathroom for a full month!

Now, if Spencer has to be admitted to the hospital, well that's an additional cost of course.

If it's no trouble, please send an additional five or six minivans.

Thanks,

Steve

Free Parking

Seattle Children's Hospital has free parking!

And for $500, you can chat with a doctor. Which is exactly what we did. Of course, we were a bit late for the appointment, not so much because of the long line at the border, the treacherous weather, or the hideous traffic, but because of the outlet malls and the cheap US dollar.

Spencer found that nurses are universal. Always pleasant, caring, and professional of course, but more than anything they have an overwhelming compulsion to take height, weight, blood pressure and temperature. So they did.

Dr. Park is a specialist in neuroblastoma. We went to pick her brains about the various trials that are going on in the field and get an opinion on what would be good for Spencer. Our hospital had already sent down all his scans and clinical summary. Armed with that knowledge, plus up-to-the minute height, weight, blood pressure, and temperature, we were ready to begin.

We discussed four different clinical trials and matched them up against where Spencer is at and what our goals as a family are. Three of the trials are offered at Seattle Children's. None of them are offered at BC Children's. We went through them all and discussed them without regard to where they were offered or what they cost. Tracey could provide all the technical details about why one is preferred over another; I just know what the conclusion was. It seems like ABT-751, the drug Spencer originally wrote his letter to MSP about, would be a very good place to start.

Temsirolimus might also be a good alternative. Dr. Park was not a fan of the Vermont trial for Nifurtimox for Spencer because its efficacy may be tied into joint delivery with the same chemo that Spencer has had nineteen rounds of. Zometa was a good choice to try targeting bone disease, but I think it got knocked lower down the list given the nasty things we've already done to Spencer's kidneys.

So the plan? Well, as it turns out, the ABT-751 is available off-trial at BC Children's. Tracey met with Spencer's doctor today and she agrees that this is a good thing to try. We should be able to start fairly quickly and we should know relatively quickly if it is working or not. The second choice, temsirolimus, may open up for trial in Vancouver in January. It was a really good meeting in Seattle. So even though we might end up doing exactly what we might have done without going there, it is really good to know that different minds are more or less aligned in the same direction and we are comfortable doing what is right for Spencer, not just what is inexpensive or locally available.

I was a little disappointed in the visit in that I didn't get a chance to meet anyone in the Desperate Foreign Family Cash Extraction Department. I really wanted to see them keep a straight face and tell me that it was necessary to spend $80,000 for tests and infusion costs to go along with a free drug trial. If we do ever end up in Seattle for trials, Dr. Park seems more than willing to work with our hospital to keep costs to a minimum.

Over the last five years, we've paid over $3000 to park at BC Children's Hospital. Somehow, I think free parking isn't as cheap as we might think.

Larousse de Poche and Other Biblical Stories

Canadians have a fear of being trapped outside the country with a serious medical condition. We're conditioned that way since birth. So it was a bit alarming.

A fortuitous set of circumstances found us charged with the responsibility of having family fun. The boys had their choice of anything and decided upon a weekend away in fancy hotel with a pool and shopping — in Seattle.

The medicals went to work. They are all about fun. They set about optimizing the platelet levels so Spencer would have a good chance of keeping the blood inside his vessels. After a recreational top-up on Friday afternoon, we were good to go.

Everything went well. There was Target and Best Buy and Costco and a whole raft of fancy shops in Bellevue Square. I found Boater's World just down the street. We even went up the Space Needle and ordered lattes and hot chocolate.

Our friends Al, Sue and Hadley dropped by the hotel and we all swam in the pool. I think Spencer and Hadley were impressed that an entire U13 girls soccer team arrived for a swim while we were there, but they pretended not to notice. We all went upstairs and ordered desserts from room service.

Then it happened: The medical thing that Canadians fear when they are in a foreign country. It was like all of a sudden it appeared — a lump that was completely unnoticed before. I was scared senseless.

"Al, you're an ear nose and thumb doctor aren't you? What do you think this is?" I showed him my thumb. It had a tumor growing out of the knuckle. It had been in pain for some time, but the bump was new and growing fast.

Al poked and prodded and then pulled out his iPhone to do a little web research. Soon he was ready with a diagnosis. "It's a ganglionic cyst," he declared, "no doubt caused by excessive Blackberry use." Treatment options included needle aspiration (high rate of recurrence) or surgical excision. Google turned up a more radical folk-oriented remedy now frowned upon by the medical community: whack it with a book.

That sounded good to me. A solution in line with a Canadian medical budget. I seized a copy of the Holy Bible and prepared to whack my thumb. "Wait! You can't do that yourself," Al said. Yet he wasn't jumping off the bed to help me. He may have had an issue with whacking a friend with a Bible, New Testament and everything, smack in the middle of Hanukkah. More likely just a bad feeling about what might happen to his malpractice insurance rates if this went badly wrong. Maybe it was that 'first do no harm' thing. "You should really wait until you're back inside a country with full health coverage."

It was hard to fault his logic. I put the Bible down. Yesterday was more room service and shopping and the return trip home. We all had a great time and it was a really, really fun get away. We told our usual lies to the border people and re-entered Canada with our loot and no mortgage on our home held by a Seattle medical center.

As we were finishing dinner tonight, I put my thumb up on the table and we began talking about what to do. Foster wasted no time and grabbed a handy copy of Larousse de Poche 2006 – a two-inch thick French dictionary. Tracey suggested I should lay my hand flat, but if I rotated the thumb the ganglionic cyst stuck straight up, which appeared to be a better angle. I thought we were still in the conceptual phase.

Foster was way past the concept stage.

Whack!

I was stunned. The pain was intense. The evil grin on Foster's face was shocking. Then I looked at my thumb and the hard lump was gone. Foster had cured me. He is a master healer and my hero. Now we just have to make sure he doesn't start chasing Spencer around with a copy of Larousse de Poche. The platelets are a bit low again.

A Twelve-Year-Old Vampire Says Thanks

My name is Spencer Dolling and I am a twelve-year-old vampire who lives in Port Coquitlam. I have been fighting a cancer called stage 4 neuroblastoma for six years. The treatment that I have affects my bone marrow and I need lots of blood transfusions. I have had around 300 blood transfusions in six years. This came from 450 different donors.

Out of the 300 transfusions, about 110 have been platelets. Platelets are blood cells that help with clotting to stop bleeding. During all my years in treatment, my bone marrow has become weak and this year in particular, I needed about fifty platelet transfusions.

The other kind of blood I get is called packed red blood cells. It contains hemoglobin that carries oxygen. If your blood does not contain enough hemoglobin, you can barely climb a flight of stairs and you will look very pale.

A couple of months ago, I went over to the Canadian Blood Services clinic on Oak Street to see how they got blood from people. I found that it takes about an hour to donate whole blood. The whole blood is later divided into red cells, plasma and platelets for different patients. Whole blood can be stored for several weeks. If they do not have the type of blood that you need, they can get it from another province.

Some people just donate platelets. A special machine uses apheresis that picks the platelets out of your blood and then gives the other unused blood back to you. It takes about two hours to donate platelets. Platelets can be only kept for five days.

I also found out that the people who donate blood come quite often and spend lots of their free time giving. I had never thought about it before but I now wonder what they get in return. I decided to make them a Christmas card to thank them. I mean really, if you think about it, they've saved my life only about 300 times.

Canadian Blood Services in BC gets about 110,000 blood units donated a year. At this time of year people are really busy and sometimes forget the need for blood in the blood bank. This year over the holidays they will need an extra 1,200 units of blood donated to meet BC's needs. I think that we forget that blood isn't just used for car accidents or surgeries. It is used a lot for cancer patients like myself.

Blood is really important to me and my family so I can do simple things like go to school, play outside, or just stay out of the hospital. Maybe I'm not really a vampire, but I would like to thank the people who give their time to donate blood and even those who are now thinking about it.

A Shot of Flu and a Shot in the Arm

A strain of it killed more people during World War One than all the bombs and bullets combined, but that doesn't mean that this year's flu is dangerous. Well, except maybe to the elderly and those with weak immune systems. That's why Spencer got a flu shot this year.

So naturally, he's in the hospital with the influenza A.

Spencer seems to be doing better. He's not barking like a small seal being kicked by a donkey any more. His fevers are less intense. It's kind of nice to have something else to blame fevers on.

I think I had it last week, but it only bothered me for a couple of days. Flu shots are a wonderful thing. Some ABT-751 got shipped this week. I would like to think that Abbott would have shipped it anyway, but I don't think receiving this letter slowed them down any. In fairness, they were dealing with a safety issue, which they had to clear up. Spencer didn't have any obligation to be fair. They only refer to him as SBD and his name gets ***** out in correspondence.

> Dear ****************
>
> My name is ******* ******* or SD. I'm pretty sure you know who I am. I am a twelve-year-old boy from Vancouver. I have had stage four neuroblastoma for five and a bit years. I have had two bone marrow

transplants, full body radiation and lots and lots of chemotherapy. My bone marrow has gotten very weak from all that so I am very platelet deficient. We were looking for a different chemo to start that didn't affect my platelets as much so we stumbled across ABT-751. We also had heard someone talking about and it looked really good because it didn't affect my platelets and it had mild side effects. So we thought we would see who had it on study (this is around October). We found out that the only places that had it on study close to us were Seattle, Toronto and Quebec. We did not really want to go to Toronto or Quebec because it was Christmas and we didn't want to be so far from our family so it had to be Seattle. It turned out that Seattle was way too pricey and unreasonable. Then one of the doctors found it off study made by Abbott and they could send it to Vancouver then they could give it to me at the hospital. We ordered it around December 1st and they said it would be here a few weeks before Christmas. It didn't come. They said because the shipping companies are so busy before Christmas and that a lot of their staff are on holidays so they would have to ship it later and it would arrive a few days after New Year's. We were fine with that so they gave me a different chemo to stop me from having pain in my back. We waited and waited. Now it's January 9 and I'm wondering if you will actually send it. Now I am having to have more chemo to stop my back pain and fevers.

I don't know who you are or what exactly you do but I do know that you work at Abbott. It may not be you but someone is getting my hopes up then letting them fall off a mountain. It may not even be someone that works at Abbott, it may just be someone who works for the Government of Canada or the United States, but someone is doing it and I want to know why in the world it is taking so long to get something that they said would take two weeks to get. I understand that it's not licensed in Canada but it's been five and a bit weeks so I'm still wondering where's my ABT-751. All I'm saying is please hurry and send it so maybe it will help the pain in my back from my cancer.

PS: I know you like to use little stars so I thought I'd use them too ****************

Thanks From ******* ******* or SD

Now Spencer is going to have to work on his backlog of thank you letters.

Assumptions

It's been a while since the last update. People generally assume that things must be going well and we're too busy living life to be bothered writing.

I wish that were the case. It's been a difficult few weeks.

Spencer has been in a lot of pain the last few weeks. The bump on his head disappeared, which was nice. No radiation required. Maybe the ABT is doing good things. But he has other pains pop up in his hips, back, knee, and ribs. He's been taking a lot of narcotics and just trying to be comfortable. I suppose the good news is that they he doesn't have persistent pain in one spot. But pain is pain and it's not fun.

He hasn't been to school. He missed the public speaking assignment in class, but he did deliver his vampire speech to the first and second year medical students who were kicking off their blood drive – about 500 of them, some in person and others by video conference in remote cities. Nobody told him he should be nervous, so he wasn't. It was great. I have had reasonable luck with backgammon. I think I win half the games. But it doesn't matter how big the dose of narcotics, I still can't win at Guitar Hero.

Against the Current

It's been a while since the last update. People generally assume that things are going badly and the updates must be difficult.

That's not the case. It's been a pretty good couple of weeks. No news is no news.

There was the pain thing of course. It was intense in Spencer's knee. We thought it might be disease, or maybe neuropathy from the ABT. It seems like maybe it wasn't either of those things. It might have been a steroid he was on to stimulate appetite. Whatever it was, the pain went away.

Sometimes it's best not to ask too many questions. Tracey is courageous. She sensed a window of opportunity. I believe the tickets were booked and paid for before we actually got an answer from Spencer's oncologist whether or not it was a good idea. We are going to Mexico. I put in my vacation request. It was rather more like a terrorist demand than a vacation request. Choice is only an illusion anyway.

The four-year-old salmon can choose if he wants to swim up the river.

We went sailing on Sunday. Scupper stayed home, but Graeme, our new nephew, came for his first sail. I think he liked it best when the engine was running.

Spectacular. Then, Sunday night, a lot of blood. Very scary. Tracey and Spencer headed for the hospital. Foster and I stayed home.

But there was good news. I beat Guitar Hero. I battled Lou and I won. Now I'm technically on the same level as Spencer and Foster, although I don't have five stars on any of my songs, and I've never even played a song on medium yet.

Oh yes, and the bleeding. Tracey and Spencer never came home. I went to visit them on Monday morning. Spencer's doctor and nurse were there. Most of the conversation seemed to be centered on Mexico and making sure that we have a letter explaining the bag full of narcotics we plan to take. There was very little concern around the fact that Spencer was in the hospital getting transfusions of platelets and red cells two weeks before departure. Everyone was happy with the idea of a recreational transfusion the day before we go, just to be sure. And so he was discharged. Right then. Off we go.

Does the salmon worry? I think not.

We're on a mission.

Continuing Education

Tracey went downtown to the conference today to catch up with old classmates and colleagues and take in some lectures to keep her continuing education current.

Somehow, I think it was me who got the education today.

I'm glad Spencer slept until 11:00. It gave me four hours to figure out what medications he was supposed to take. I never was able to figure out exactly what I'm supposed to do to get him to eat and drink. Maybe that's a more advanced lesson.

I was able to pick up a few credits in the emergency medicine curriculum. When you call into the hospital and explain that Spencer has tightness in his chest and discomfort breathing, they want to see him.

So we drove into emergency. I went fast. Not so much because we were in a hurry, but because I figure if I'm ever going to talk my way out of a speeding ticket, nothing could work better than, "Oh, sorry about that, I'll try to slow down, it's just that my son is having trouble breathing and I need to get him to Children's Hospital."

Spencer has Triple Platinum Elite Club Status at Children's ER. There's a room full of people waiting and we get whisked in to a freshly cleaned room of our own in no time.

He got the full going over. Poking and prodding, EKGs and blood-work. Chest X-ray for giggles. I have to say I was a little disappointed. I thought maybe with electrodes being stuck all over him, I'd be able to pick up a few backgammon wins with the distraction. It didn't work that way. I got my butt kicked.

Anyway, the chest tightness remains a bit of a mystery. I'm not sure what exactly I learned other than it's more difficult in the role of responsible parent. Tracey can have it back any time she wants. We did manage to make it home in time to catch the last few minutes of the hockey game, in high definition no less. I did figure out the evening meds. It was nice to see Spencer eat a meal, even if was just pills.

Back from Mexico

t's illegal in Canada to drive a personal watercraft if you are twelve years old. That's why Mexico was created.

At least you might think that if you saw the smile on Spencer's face.

According to Foster, it takes seven seconds for spit to reach the ocean when parasailing.

Of course, we all went fishing. Next time we vow to go catching. But we did find a couple of scuba divers floating near a breaking reef — and their boat adrift about a mile away. Still, catching a barracuda would have been better.

I'm pretty sure that the doctors wouldn't want to know about jumping off cliffs into the cool fresh water of cenotes given we will also be talking about large amounts of narcotics taken for back pain, so we just won't mention it to them.

I think it was a good thing that it was Foster that fell out of the tree and had the bruising all up his side from the impact with the water. Spencer arrived home with low platelets and didn't really have enough left over for falling out of trees. We had a couple of other casualties. One of the two-way radios fell overboard while we were tacking, and the wheelchair we borrowed from the Red Cross shot out the side of the resort shuttle as we went around the corner. There were gasps of horror from the fellow passengers until they realized that the wheelchair was unoccupied as it took to its new slightly bent form.

Tracey threw a birthday party for me while we were there. No less than eighteen people! Complete with a Mr. Steve cake; it was an impressive affair.

Scupper hung out with his brother for the duration. He was reported to be very well behaved and a "good dog". I find it hard to believe, but I'm not sure why Sheila would lie to us. Perhaps he is just good in a relative sense compared to his brother Ben. Maybe Sheila was just being kind.

We missed Scupper, but we did get to visit with his friend Boston down in Puerto Morelos. Boston and Sarah are doing well and seem to know everybody in town. And a cool town it is. Just hanging there for a day makes you realize how absurd it is to associate all the wealth and technology and pace of life that we have with happiness. I'm not sure there is any relationship.

Better to live life slowly with a lot of friends than fast with a lot of money.

An Episode of House

A work friend once asked me if I had ever seen the show *House*. I hadn't. He explained it to me and said I reminded him of House. I felt flattered that I was compared to some intelligent doctor character. It wasn't until I saw the show that I realized the option remains open for comparison to an asshole with poor social skills. I must remember to ask him exactly what he meant.

Today was like an episode of *House*.

Before the drama, I should back up a bit. People ask, "How was Mexico?" I hesitate before answering and then I tell them it was really good, which is true, but there are different ways to get to really good. Really good can be fourteen days of really good, or it can be some blend of absolute excellence with some real crap. Sometimes both can be combined into the same hour.

There were a few days when Spencer was really feeling like crap. He had intense pain in his back and he was maxed out on tramadol and methadone. We could hardly get him to eat or drink anything and on a couple of occasions I had to pull the string out of the waistband of my shorts to hang IV bags from the picture frame in the hotel room while Tracey rigged all the lines and stuck needles in our boy. So if I tell people about the challenging bits, they feel so sorry for our suffering. If I only talk about Spencer riding jet skis, cliff jumping in cenotes, snorkeling, fishing, sailing, and playing backgammon in the shade, they get some idea of a sublime time in paradise. Neither image is entirely correct. If we just throw it all in the blender like a coco-banana, it all turns out pretty damn good, which is exactly what it was.

The return from paradise has been more challenging. The eating and drinking problems have continued. The pain is gone, but there is something much more deeply disturbing. It started on the plane ride home. Spencer has had some rather serious confusion and has become obsessed with certain things. His cognitive processing is spotty. When we were riding home from the airport, he started taking notes in his iPod and insisted on capturing his thoughts before he forgot things. He spent two hours writing notes. In the end, he captured about five different sentences. This from the kid who delivers speeches at medical schools.

Last night he wanted to watch the hockey game. "But the hockey game is tomorrow, Spencer."

"I know," he says, and a few seconds later, "Let's watch the hockey game." He spent forty-five minutes entering channel 22 on the remote and surprised himself every time when the world billiard championship came on instead of the Canuck's game. The episodes came and went.

Spencer went for an MRI yesterday. They were looking at his brain, checking for signs of neuroblastoma. Fortunately, his MRI came back clean. Thus, the *House* episode began in earnest. The easy diagnosis was ruled out. Sharp diagnostic minds went to work. Of course, if you are going to have good drama, you can't just have a group of doctors chattering away, the case has to get more complicated and urgent. So this morning Spencer went for the high heart rate and extreme tiredness and weakness.

The ambulance came around nine. They didn't want to take Spencer to Children's, only Eagle Ridge. Tracey told them fine, she would drive him to the edge of Vancouver and call another ambulance.

Nobody messes with Tracey. They drove Spencer to Children's.

Various experts came by to chat. Everything was potentially relevant. No detail was overlooked. Maybe the pressure on the airplane. What did we do in Mexico? Was anybody else sick? There was a lot of interest in what drugs were taken in what dosages at what times. We are at the maximum of methadone on what days and when exactly did we notice the first symptoms, etc., etc. We told them everything.

At one point, there was a psychologist and one of the freaky pain service guys who were asking a lot of questions. I came clean: "I was operating at half the maximum dose of rum and coke for the whole two weeks." I wasn't sure if it was relevant but felt compelled to disclose.

"How do you know what the maximum is?" the freaky pain service guy asked me.

"Maximum is face down in the sand," I explained. "I was nowhere near that."

"You know that is exactly how they do anesthetics — they call it the L50 dose. L is lethal so they give you half the lethal dose. There's years and years of data." This is why I find the pain service guys freaky.

In six years, Spencer has had some complicated medical issues and done some risky things, but really nothing has been terribly mysterious. He has never really generated large amounts of medical interest. Okay, maybe his second transplant, but largely he's never really stumped anyone.

The ridiculously simple single drug treatment with instantaneous results was identified. It was administered to the patient. Miraculously, his symptoms disappeared. His mind was cleared. All was well. Just a bit of Tramadol withdrawal-induced psychosis. More drugs and the addict is cured.

Of course, unlike TV, there is still the grimy business of regaining strength and getting some nutrition (NG tube tomorrow).

We need to see if all remains well, but so far so good. And there remains that nasty cancer thing; so next week there will be scans and bone marrow biopsies and whatnot to see where that is. What has the ABT done?

Rough Going

Spencer is very sick. He is quite weak and has been getting his nutrition through a feeding tube. He has had quite a bit of pain from his shingles and is still on large doses of Tramadol with the occasional hit of methadone. He has had some good days and some not so good days.

His scan results were mixed. His MIBG scan seemed to be worse than the last one with much of his liver lighting up. This is obviously a big concern. At present, they're not sure if it is a fungal infection or neuroblastoma in his liver. His bone scan has improved a good deal since January. So when Spencer says the ABT is working, he may know what he is talking about. Today he had a liver biopsy to investigate what they are seeing on the scan. If it's a fungal infection, they will use an anti-fungal drug to treat it.

If it's NB, that's not very good news and they'll try more chemo. He also had a bone marrow biopsy today. None of these biopsies does anything particularly good for Spencer, so he asked to have a couple of warts fixed. If you're going to have anesthesia, might as well have some tangible good come from it!

Tonight he is feeling good and very hungry after not being able to eat all day with the surgeries. He has managed to put on some weight and is a lot stronger today than yesterday.

We'll see what tomorrow brings.

Dr. Andrucson

It was six years and three days ago. Our regular doctor said not to worry, take some Tylenol. Tracey finally found a doctor in a walk-in clinic who took the time and listened to her when she said there was something wrong with Spencer. He was an older doctor. He moved at a different pace, and he was thorough and he took his time. He found a mass. I think we all know how the story went from there.

We found a new family doctor!

Five years, three hundred sixty four days ago, we celebrated Tracey's birthday at Children's Hospital.

I didn't get to see Spencer today. Foster had a sore throat. I woke up with a sore throat. So I left the hospital before Spencer woke up and Foster and I hung out in misery, except for the part when we went to the mall to look for new rollerblades. Then we remembered that it was Mom's birthday tomorrow and we found a black leather purse that's sort of backpack like. We did it all on our own without any help, so we know she'd love it. But just in case, we put the gift receipt inside.

Today, Spencer was in pain. Excruciating, uncontrollable pain in his shoulder and his ribs. He couldn't even talk. He had to write instructions to tell people to shut up, get out of the room, stop asking about his pain, and turn a movie on so he could change his focus. Then he wrote a new pain plan for the doctors explaining which drugs at what quantities and what times for what sorts of pain are most effective.

I think that they were listening, but I'm not sure. I wasn't there. Foster and I were at the doctor's appointment that Tracey booked for us to have our sore throats looked at. It wouldn't do to expose Spencer to something nasty while his immune system is suppressed from the chemo, and the regular family doctor wasn't there. There was an old doctor filling in. Dr. Andrucson. He asked why the older son's immune system was suppressed, and we answered. He asked what the older son's name was, and we told him. He remembered Spencer and he remembered finding a mass. And he took his time: Nearly an hour to swab a couple throats and look in ears and noses. We didn't mind waiting. We have all the time in the world for Dr. Andrucson.

Tomorrow, we'll celebrate another of Tracey's birthdays at Children's Hospital, but maybe Foster and I will wear masks. It takes a few days to get results from the swabs.

Enlightenment

Tracey picked up a book by His Holiness the Dalai Lama at Costco a few months ago. It was $8.99.

I didn't really have the attention span for it, but skimmed parts of it, picking out the good bits as it were. The thing that struck me was the whole Buddhist notion of enlightenment. I think at first, I didn't get it entirely right.

I sought insight, and for that you need high definition. If you want high definition, you need 1080 lines and progressive scan. With a decent contrast ratio and a signal source, preferably something that plays a Blu-ray disc.

So it was that the 46" LCD came into our home, and I watched *Planet Earth* in full 1080p with surround sound. And so it was.

I wondered how many Tibetan monks had 46" Sonys, and how many of them were attempting to achieve enlightenment without the right equipment.

Yet still I didn't feel enlightened, and so I skimmed a few more chapters. I recognized the need to simplify and concentrate and bring things down to their essence. The complication of it all was darkening my pending enlightenment.

I needed to quiet the lake. You can't quiet the lake when you have three different remotes. Simply programming one remote to work like three just knocks the tips off the waves. Thus, the new Logitech smart remote. And so it is with a few hours of programming, I can now press a single button (well two, really) and choose whether to watch a hockey game or switch over to play Guitar Hero. The thing even talks to the TV, the cable box, and the receiver and figures out everything. I can feel the stillness.

Now the lake is quiet, and I know I'm nearly there.

Scupper Triumphs

The epic battle is lost. Scupper wins.

I didn't realize it, but it was really a siege. For years, the enemy has been in waiting in my very presence, and slowly, slowly, slowly we've been worn down. At long last, we are conquered. I didn't even know about it until the next day.

Tracey came to the hospital and told me that she woke up in the middle of the night after a fitful sleep. And the hairy beast was in the bed. In my spot. Not quite with his head on my pillow.

Spooning her.

Worse—and this was how we know it's all over—she didn't throw him out.

Fly the flags at half-mast. I can't say that I blame Scupper. My friend Alistair came over on the weekend. We decided to get liquored up on Saturday night and cut Scupper's hair. Understand, it's not that we got liquored up and made a bad decision. It was all premeditated. We had to fix the Balding for Dollars work of the week before. Scupper looked like a fat Schnauzer that had had its head stepped on. By the first glass of wine, we had already decided we go with the East Kootenay Badger cut. Unfortunately, it all went wrong and he ended up with a quarter inch of hair everywhere. Everywhere except the scrotal area. Scupper and I have an agreement that supersedes anything I've had to drink. We just leave a ball of hair there. That way I don't accidentally cut some loose skin that might be hanging down, and he can go out in the dog world and keep the bitches guessing.

Spencer has been coming home for a few hours every evening. His infection is slowly getting better. His biggest issue (other than that little cancer problem) is weaning off the pain medications. He's been a bit quiet of late from all the drugs. Although today we played our first backgammon in about a month. Two games. He won them both. It was just luck. Three sets of doubles in a row.

Tomorrow, we are going to check out a go-kart track. There is an indoor one in Richmond that is apparently very fast. The plan is to have his birthday party there on Wednesday, so tomorrow is the trial run to make sure he'll have fun. Spencer might be half an inch short of the height requirement. I think we'll just show the bald head and say that it's not fair kids with hair are taller. With the hair issue as a distraction, the topic of whether or not it's safe to drive under the influence of a massive load of narcotics won't come up.

It Feels Faster When You're Slung Low

Blondie was driving Race 2. I was up above taking pictures. I heard a whump and looked down to see Yoshi bouncing off the wall. My first thought was, "Oh, oh, he's run out of steam." He qualified seven seconds slower than Bowser. I thought maybe there was too much methadone and Tramadol and was just time to call it a day and have a rest.

But I watched as Yoshi took off. He hadn't under-steered and missed the corner; he'd done a four-wheel drift and slammed in sideways. I watched him through the next three turns and he was definitely not slowing down. He was reeling in Toad and Frying Pan. He came back down the straightaway and I saw the look.

I haven't seen the look in a long time. Mostly I see the methadone look. The quiet boy without emotion. The blank stare. It's better than the pain look, but it's nothing like this one. This was the animated look. This was the "get the hell out of my way I have a world to conquer" look. It's a look a little more directly connected to the soul. Sort of fear and determination packaged together. It can't be generated playing video games, no matter how good the graphics. It was a look that was good for Bowser's soul.

I had plans to handicap the race. I talked to the pain docs this morning and asked how much methadone I should give to the other kids to make the race fair. They suggested that if I gave everybody the same dose Spencer was on, they wouldn't be able to drive at all.

So we did the handicapping based on the times in the qualifying race instead. Funny thing was, by the third race Yoshi had picked up his seven seconds. All of the near teenagers were within a second of each other, so Yoshi kicked butt on corrected time. Waluigi won on the uncorrected time (Happy Birthday, Jared). Mario got the drift award (well done, Foster).

Of course, Blondie beat them all, but she wasn't eligible for prizes. We might have to go back on Monday, Spencer's actual birthday, because the first race is free. Of course, Bowser would do anything to see the look again. And then, just like in some epic endurance race, we had to help him out of the car and send him off to be hooked up to an IV (after cake and pizza of course).

Mother's Day

I didn't have a chance to update yesterday because the server was down at the hospital.

Spencer had his surgery yesterday. They cleaned out his infection. Nothing too complicated and it went well.

There's a small problem today: They left a dressing packed in the wound. Imagine a half-inch hole in your lower back that goes through to the hip bone, packed with cotton. That's kind of what Spencer has, but they don't actually use cotton. The surgeon came by to "unpack" it today. Pain was the problem.

I say small problem. I think Spencer would disagree. Okay, it was a major problem. It was too painful and the cocktail of painkillers hadn't set in enough, so the surgeon went away and suggested Spencer or the nurse could pull it out whenever he was comfortable.

A little while later, they decided to have a go since Spencer was already drugged up. Tracey attached the clamp. Spencer did the pulling.

Imagine pulling a bullet out of your own back. A big one, say .45 calibre.

Needless to say, we enjoyed a nice glass of the Mother's Day sparkling shiraz in the playroom with the lovely meal that Uncle Johnny brought. Happy Mother's Day! I hope you all got to spend quality time with your kids like Tracey did today.

Spencer has also been enjoying his birthday presents a little early. He pooled together a little of his own fun money and Nanny Pop birthday money with a Mom and Dad contribution to get a 32" flat screen TV. Foster got him the new Mario Kart for Wii game and so the real Yoshi and Mario have been racing in full color in the hospital room. Why wait? I hope he still has some fun tomorrow. Maybe we'll be able to go home soon and mount his new TV on the wall in his room.

Teenager at Last

Spencer and I spent a couple of hours on his birthday working on one of those complex Lego models. I haven't seen that kind of concentration in weeks. They must have his drugs about right, which probably means it's time to mess with them.

He had an uncomfortable time yesterday. Things don't feel right in his belly and he has had pain return to his knee and elbow. The ultrasound shows he has some fluid buildup in his abdomen and lungs and his liver is a bit larger than it was. The lesions inside his liver look a bit fuzzier. There are no more of them and they are not bigger, so that is not bad news.

The bullet hole in his hip is healing up well. They've determined that the infection is e-coli and it will take several more weeks of antibiotics to drive it out of his bone.

Today he will start another round of chemo. Hopefully, he'll be feeling more comfortable soon.

Forgive Me if I am Not Miserable

Sheila and Suzanne got a bit of grief today. Sheila is Spencer's oncologist. Suzanne is his primary nurse. Together they know us as a family at least as well as, well, our family. They are family. We make all our important decisions together.

Today, there was a meeting among the medical staff about Spencer. Some concern was expressed that perhaps unwarranted hope was being passed on to us by pressing ahead with chemo when there is really no reason to be hopeful. There was also some alarm that we seem to walk around the hallways smiling and generally cheerful. It was observed that I am quiet. I guess the overriding concern, whether stated or not, was whether Tracey and I are at all plugged into reality or if we wander about in a serious state of denial.

Forgive me if I am not miserable.

Believe me, I am miserable, but I've had six years of training. I fake it well.

A long time ago, Spencer was statistically dead. That is to say, the likelihood of attending his wedding was infinitesimally small. The likelihood of him ever being a teenager was tiny. Problem was, we had this vibrant, very much alive, little boy to contend with. We had choices to make. We had to decide if every day Spencer was a little closer to death, or if every day he was alive and we should damn well live the best we can. If it's not obvious which choice we made, then we have failed.

We might very well be on a train headed down the tracks with the bridge washed out. We do of course have the choice. Shall we run to the back of the train, hide underneath a seat, and moan and whimper, or would it be better to get dressed for dinner, head to the dining car, and have a few cocktails while enjoying the scenery? If we could jump off the train, believe me we would. In the meantime, have you seen my dinner jacket?

So if you see me hopeful about the chemo my son is getting, don't worry. I'm under no illusion that all of a sudden things will be better and remission is just around the corner. I don't believe that any more than anyone else. Trust me, I do the mental processing twenty-four hours a day. Do I believe the chemo might relieve his pain and make him feel better, and maybe we can go home to have some fun or get another pass and go go-karting or whatever? Absolutely. It is possible.

I also understand that we are not waiting for God's gentle hand to guide him to a better place. Neuroblastoma is an ugly beast that will rip apart his body with painful tumors. So let's look at the alternatives. Being treated to death is not the worst thing that can happen.

So no, we haven't crushed Spencer's hopes and told him he is dying. Last time I checked, he was alive. I think they call that living. Will we come to that point? Yes. Likely. We discuss it every day or so. Have we taken advantage of all the wonderful palliative services that are available to us? No. Thanks. We're comfortable for now on 3B with the people Spencer knows giving him the care that he is familiar with. We don't need to get freaky and fill our house with hospital equipment or go and live at Canuck Place. Maybe later. Not now. And don't ask, we know it's there for us if we need it.

So suck it up. Get over it. The Dollings aren't crazy. Their heads are screwed on tighter than yours. We've got a job to do. Let's head for the dining car.

Checking Out

We had checked in a couple of weeks before. Of course, we had been regulars off and on for six years.

Foster and I played with Scupper down in the parking garage. It was a way to blow off a little steam. I couldn't really do a full arm extension on the ball chucker with the low overhead, so I had to throw side arm with somewhat reduced accuracy. Foster was short enough that he could get a full overhead swing, but he tended to be a bit wild just the same. Scupper really didn't mind where the ball went as long as he could chase it.

It was good for Scupper to have a little run around and get some attention and exercise. He's had too many hours alone in the truck. Skidding on the concrete helps to keep his nails trimmed without the yelping and the blood that sometimes spills when I do it with the clippers.

We knew it was time to stop when a hard shot bounced squarely into the driver's door of a parked Audi. The slimy tennis ball left a dirty imprint on an otherwise immaculate black paint job. We hoped there wasn't a dent, but we didn't really bother to check. It was time to go upstairs. We locked Scupper back in the truck. There would be no sneaking him in this time.

The little paper cup of chardonnay I had been nursing was still there. It was warm. I had been giving them a hard time at the front desk in recent days. If they weren't going to get me a wine cooler for the room, all I asked for was a plug for the sink so that the little ice chips wouldn't all melt down the drain before my wine was properly chilled. They seldom take my requests seriously. Always, they have higher priorities.

Tracey was with Spencer in the room. It was supposed to be Tracey's night off, but Spencer asked me to call her in. He'd never done that before. So she came with Foster and we were all together for a change.

The room was a little more crowded. The respiratory therapist had arrived. She was fitting Spencer with an oxygen mask with little purple eyes and whiskers. The mask was kind of young looking for a thirteen year old, but I guess that's all they have at a children's hospital. Spencer didn't really notice. He was starting to have trouble talking. He took big gulps of the oxygen.

We were old hands at the medical arts, but this was all new for us. Six years of more or less continuous treatment including chemotherapy, radiation, bone marrow transplants, surgeries and drug therapies and you would think we would have seen it all by now. But we had never seen Spencer this sick.

Five weeks before, Spencer had been piloting jet skis and swimming in underground caves in Mexico. Now the little spots of neuroblastoma weren't just abstractions on the nuclear medicine scans waiting to be targeted by the latest treatment. Instead, they were all too real, eating away his liver, resistant to any more treatment. His lungs were filling with fluid. He was slowly drowning, and a lifejacket would do nothing for him.

The resident dropped by, all serious. She was checking on Spencer, listening to his lungs. I had to ask her an important question, "Do you drive a black Audi?"

"No," she replied, "Why do you ask?"

"Never mind. It's not important."

She asked me to join her outside for a private conversation. We sat down in the little meeting room on the ward. She seemed upset and a little uncertain how to continue. Somehow, the burden fell on me to be the calm and collected one even though I really felt like I should be screaming and banging my head against the wall. But I did feel calm. She eventually asked if we wanted to move Spencer downstairs to the intensive care unit and hook him up to a ventilator to help him breathe.

"Would that make Spencer more comfortable?" I asked. "What would we gain?"

"The ventilator can be quite stressful for kids sometimes. It can be frightening. We would sedate him. It is not always comfortable, but it might give you some more time. Hours. Maybe a day or so at most."

"What is the alternative?"

"We can keep him here on 3B and give him morphine to keep him comfortable. Though the morphine will slow his breathing." The implications didn't require explanation. A death spiral with no hyperbole.

I am sure it would have been easier for the staff if we had just transferred down to the ICU, but we were comfortable having the family together in the care of the medical team we knew upstairs. All we could do was what we thought was best for Spencer and convince ourselves that we hadn't made a pact to kill him with morphine.

We killed him with morphine.

Though I am sure there are medical ethicists who could guide me through a more enlightened exploration with far less judgmental terminology, I don't need it. There is no guilt. No blame. No need to explain.

At every moment of Spencer's life, right up to the very last moment, we did what was right for him and kept him comfortable.

We didn't kill him with morphine.

We kept him comfortable, just one step ahead of the processes in his body over which we had no control. He took slow raspy breaths.

Foster cried uncontrollably.

The morphine took away any anxiety for Spencer. The intervals between his breaths stretched out as the hours went by. We hugged. We cried. We said goodbye without speaking.

Until the last interval was infinite.

There is a little room at the end of the ward called the "Quiet Room". Usually it's great place to sneak through and have a pee in the ensuite bathroom when the other ones are occupied. For years, I had walked by the comfy couch and the tables with bibles and grieving literature and it was all too apparent what the real purpose of the Quiet Room was. They have a damn room for it. Wine coolers aside, they think of everything.

The Quiet Room is where families go to cry until they run out of tears. Which takes surprisingly less time than might be imagined. There was no particular need to pull ourselves together. We probably could have stayed there for days and nobody would have bothered us. But we did pull ourselves together, and laughed and shared memories. As dawn broke, we made the first phone call on the conveniently provided phone.

We discovered that the tear reservoirs are refillable. Perhaps even infinite.

Someone asked me once what it was like to live all these years with the cancer. I explained that it's a bit like having a terrorist threaten to kill your kid. It could happen any day when you aren't expecting it. Still you send them out to play, and every now and then you hear gunshots on the playground to remind you of the credibility of the threat. The weight of that threat was now lifted, but it's like replacing leg shackles with barbed wire underwear. Go. Run. Be free!

The capacity to feel is not infinite. At some point, we just ran out of feeling. There wasn't anything left to feel. It was time to check out.

There was no real checkout procedure. Nothing to sign. No bill to pay. Just a few hugs and we walked out the door of the ward and took the elevator to the parking garage.

The Audi was gone. Scupper was there waiting for us.

When the morning shift arrived, Spencer's name was wiped off the board. A memory foam mattress and half bottle of chardonnay were the only evidence of our stay.

Damn. We forgot to leave a tip.

Remission

Re-mis-sion: 1) a period during which the symptoms of a disease are abated 2) the part of the story where Spencer is dead, and the rest of the family packs up the house and sails away

Train Wreck

So here we are now among the tangled mess of broken cars. Welcome to our train wreck!

Tracey and I have been deeply moved by all the words of sympathy that have poured out on the website, over the phone and through email. I know people agonize over what to say and how to say it, but it really doesn't matter. It really is the thought that counts and we appreciate the thought. It's tough.

We were all laughing and telling jokes by 5:00 am yesterday. Then we made the first phone calls and completely fell apart. Back and forth it went all day. I told friends that we were going to have to make decisions about arrangements because people would need to time to make their costumes. That triggered nervous laughter. We haven't made arrangements yet. We will meet with the funeral home tomorrow.

It's tough. When you have a wedding, you might agonize over whom to invite, but at the end of the day, you know how big of a venue to book. With a funeral it's so hard. I don't know that a couple of hundred seats is going to be big enough. Spencer touched many people. Plus, I think it's going to emphasize fun over sadness, so it should be a popular event. Anyway, we'll make some decisions and post notice of arrangements here tomorrow afternoon. We won't have a service until sometime mid to late next week.

We have the perfect amount of flowers already, so we will also let you know what you can do instead of sending more. Today, I was gratified by all the people that were shocked at the news of Spencer's passing. Not because it's nice to shock people, but it's so much nicer to hear than "at last his suffering is over." He really didn't suffer. The last few months have been difficult, but Spencer lived a fantastic life right to the end. And he knew it.

Spencer said it best: "Apart from my cancer, you can see that I have a fantastic life."

The Speech

If you are sitting next to a doctor, shake their hand and tell them you are honored.

If you are sitting next to a nurse, give them a hug and tell them you are in awe.

If you are a nurse, you have an odd person trying to hug you, sorry about that.

Wow. How did we end up here? We certainly didn't choose this. We had no choice at all. How is it then that the greatest lesson that Spencer taught us was that we do have a choice every hour and every day and that we can choose exactly how we want to live our lives?

If you are able, at important points in your life, to look back and say you have absolutely no regrets, it's a pretty wonderful feeling. Believe me, we know.

Spencer, "Spence", "Buddy", "Bud", "Maddy", "Nurk the All Powerful", "Penker". We miss you, buddy. We are here to honor you today.

I think though that you must have a good public relations staff. All these people here believe that you were some flawless wonderful gift to the world. I think they should know the truth.

They should understand that there are a handful of fathers in this room that would not have wanted you left alone with their daughters. You had a serious drug problem and you skipped a lot of school. And all of this before you were a teenager.

But let's start at the beginning.

I checked the log of the sailing vessel Snapdragon. May 7th, 1995, was the first mention of you in the log. Five days before you were born. You were called "Bump". We sailed with Bob and Sue that day and caught a salmon.

Your mom always hoped you would be shaped like a salmon — small pointy head, no shoulders. It didn't quite work out the way she hoped. There were thirty hours of painful laboring and then a C-section, but in the end, you were a lot cuter than a salmon-shaped baby would have been.

I remember the first night that we brought you home from the hospital. It was a very loud, long night and I was very nearly convinced that fatherhood was a huge mistake. Then your mom discovered that she could stick her little finger in your mouth you would stop wailing. Thus began thirteen years of bliss.

There was no mention of you again in the log until a full two weeks after you were born on May 27th. I remember that day. We took you to Snug Cove and we were enjoying calamari at Doc Morgan's and you had done something in your diaper that was apparently Dad's job. You were about the size of a football so I grabbed you in one arm like one, jumped over the railing and carried you that way down the dock to the boat to change your diaper. Walking back up the dock, people were staring in shocked disbelief at the sight of this father so casually carrying a precious newborn in one arm. I guess at various times throughout your life people have been in a state of shocked disbelief.

Forgive us, Spencer. There is a temptation to measure your life, and if we do it in years, the number comes up far short of what anyone can imagine as a reasonable number and that makes us sad. But when we look at it in other ways, we can't help but be happy.

You've always had a unique perspective and approach to life. You had a favorite saying; at least it was a favorite of Mom's and mine. You would say "Mom" (or "Dad"), followed by a pause, and then, "I have a question". Your questions were announced and left unposed until you had our full attention. It was like you were filling in all the pieces of the great puzzle of life and each question was important and you knew that.

We even wrote down some of your early questions. At age three, you were sitting around the dinner table and asked Mom, "Where does broccoli come from?" Mom told you that "Farmers grow it in their fields and they bring it to Safeway where we buy it." You asked, "Where do bunny rabbits come from?" Mom answered, "They come from mommy and daddy bunny rabbits." Then she asked you, "Where do you come from, Spencer?" You had already put together those pieces of life's great puzzle and had the correct answer at the tip of your tongue. "I come from Home Depot."

By age four you had everything all figured out. The log notes that we were tied up at Silva Bay enjoying a nice dinner and you asked, "After dinner can we go and walk the docks and look for girls?" But there was a dark side to all of this.

You weren't just content to enjoy the company of girls and laugh and play a game. You liked to sit next to them and gain their confidence. Then you would persuade them to take off their shoes and be comfortable. And then you would get them to take off their socks. And then you would play with their toes. More than once, a little girl came running out of your little play tent screaming, "He's trying to get me to take my socks off!" And it wasn't just the little girls. The babysitter was fair game too. Thankfully, you grew out of this one before long and it didn't seem to cause any problems later in life. At least that we know of. Logan, did Spencer ever ask you to take off your shoes?

We could measure your life by the things you've done. You've sailed boats, big ones and little ones, and traveled to Mexico and Hawaii and the Caribbean and Disneyland and Disney World. And shot arrows from a bow. Climbed walls, and caught fish. Lots and lots of fish. And read novels, thick ones. And learned to speak French. Picked out a puppy. Raised a dog. Been to camp. Flown in a helicopter. Watched killer whales hunt and dolphins play. You've caught rock cod and fed them to eagles, in flight. And built things out of wood. Swam in cool rivers. Jumped off cliffs into cenotes. Stuck everything together with hot melt glue. You've been on TV and the radio. And you've written a speech and talked to an audience of five hundred. You've met some of your heroes. Rowed a dingy. Played guitar. Skied down a mountain. Skied through a valley. Shot things out of your own cannon, mounted on your own electric assault vehicle. You've raced go-karts. Jumped on trampolines. You've played soccer and baseball. Rode a bicycle, with rollerblades on. You've been fingerprinted and thrown in a police car. Planted a garden. Built a fence. Rode in a red Ferrari. Squashed bugs. You've caught butterflies, tadpoles, caterpillars, squid, clams, octopus, jellyfish, snakes, spiders, and some really ugly lingcod and just about anything else that would take your hook or fit in your net. And you've laughed and you've cried and you've loved.

When Marilyn came over the other day to learn about you, I think she expected to help make happy a sad tale of a boy who struggled and lost a long battle with cancer, but that is not really the story. Not even close, as she learned and we have known. We hear words like courage and determination and bravery and battle and hero, and to be honest, I don't know what they mean. What I do know is that cancer was a big part of your life, and it shaped your life, and guided its course, and ultimately set its duration. But cancer never defined who you were, and we won't for a moment try and sweep it under the rug as a footnote to your life. You did everything on your own terms.

The long list of things you've done were not the result of enthusiastic parents pushing you to do things so we could check things off on your "been there, done that" list on accelerated schedule. All we could ever do was give you the opportunity. You seized it and lead us there and we never once had to push you. I don't think it ever really occurred to you that cancer was this really big thing that was supposed to slow you down, and it wasn't as though you didn't know what you were up against. You watched it take your Grandma, and your friends, Kevin and Jesstin, and especially Will. What did you have as the password on your computer? "Never give up." We never used those words. That was something inside you.

Spencer was lucky. He had an amazing mom. Tracey was his friend and companion and caregiver and chief medical researcher and advocate. She loved him and knew him and knew what he needed. She was in charge of cuddles. And there is a hospital full of people who would move Heaven and Earth to do whatever she asked for. In part because she was pretty much always right, but also because she baked cookies. She cleared the decks for anything that might be looming on the fun agenda.

. . .

They have a commonly used phrase at the clinic now: "the recreational transfusion." That's a top-up of platelets or red blood cells usually before a weekend where we plan on doing something that requires a lot of energy or has risk of bleeding, even though it is not a strict medical necessity.

We don't worry too much about the negative impact that Spencer has had on the world's supply of blood. He kind of took care of that. One day he had a question: "Where does all the blood come from?" Then based on the answer, he set about saying thank you to some donors. In understated Spencer style, things just kind of took off from there. As we speak, there is a whole cyber nation of strange orange Running Maniacs who are organizing blood drives across the country in his honor. He just had that ability to inspire people.

I guess in spite of his toe thing and the drug use and skipping school, he was a sweet kid. I remember once Tracey called me at work. Spencer was in kindergarten and had been called into the principal's office. "What did he do?" I asked. "He stuck his finger up," she said. "Stuck his finger up what?" I asked. On it went until finally I figured out that he had flipped the bird to the recess monitor. Another kid had put him up to it and Spencer didn't know what it meant.

During his interrogation, the principal asked him if he knew any bad words. "Yes," he explained, "stupid" and "shut up". That afternoon Tracey explained to him all the other bad words.

Maybe that was the point in Spencer's life where true innocence was gone forever. After diagnosis, he grew up fast, and his intelligence turned to wisdom. Wisdom is rare in a ten year old, but you could just hang out with Spencer and talk and learn a lot. You would just forget he was a kid. He was a joy to be with, even in silence.

But he did kid things. He was an expert couch potato. He played all the video games, and when they got boring, he was always creating something with his hands. He loved to play games. Skip Bo, Settlers of Catan, Risk, Monopoly, Hospitalopoly, card games, and backgammon. And Spencer was a wicked poker player.

. . .

And Spencer, you had an awesome brother. Foster is strong and sweet and caring and patient and kind. You helped teach him all these things, and they will be with him for a lifetime, along with all the memories of being with you.

And great friends. You actually managed to talk about your great friends and the love for your brother and family and publish it in the national newspaper as part of the permanent record. How special is that?

Do you know how many people never say these things and regret forever that they didn't? What a gift. Thank you, Spence, for bringing life to my iPod. Our music collection had kind of hit bottom. We knew that when the *Shrek 2* soundtrack was the best CD we had bought in years. Now at least half of the good stuff comes from you. Oh, and since I get the last word, two things: Mark Knopfler is not hillbilly music, and Roy Orbison is not a form of torture.

And now, Spencer, I think I would like to recognize a few of the individuals in your life who have made a difference. I want to single out all those who have cared for you, played with you, inspired you, driven you, taught you, and coached you. I want to recognize all the people that you have cared about. I want to list all of those who you have inspired. I want to single out the mothers who give their kids an extra hug, the runners who are going up hills saying "Never Give Up." The hockey players who think you kick ass. I want to thank each one of the people who have prayed for you individually and recognize them by name. I want spend a moment and talk about each of the people who think you are a pretty special kid who has made a difference in their lives.

Spencer, we have a problem!

I don't know where to begin, and I don't know where to end. I think perhaps there is no ending. Maybe we've stumbled across the measure of a life if indeed a life ever needed to be measured rather than just enjoyed. Let's measure it based on the space you occupy in people's hearts. Let's take the cumulative volume of all of the love that you have created. Let's use that as the measure and forget about the whole age thing. If we did convert all that to the age equivalent, I hope to live to be as old as you. You wise old soul. What a fantastic life.

We love you to infinity and beyond.

Missing You

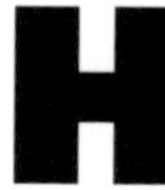ey Bud. It's been a month. We miss you terribly. Hope you're okay.

We're all doing okay. We're not quite sure how we're supposed to be doing. It seems like we should be weeping and moaning and what not, but that got old after a while.

What is staggering is the ordinariness of everything. We get up. We shower. Get dressed. Work. School. Baseball. Laundry and dirty dishes. Costco. Whatever. There doesn't seem to be an instruction manual. Is that all there is? We just get our act together and carry on?

Seems like it's a possibility.

There are other options. I've been suggesting that we should just sell the cars, the house, the boat, and just about everything and go buy a Beneteau in the Caribbean and go sailing for a few years. Mom likes the idea of going sailing, but she doesn't think we should sell the house. I suppose she's right. It might be a really dumb financial move because last time we checked, Beneteaus don't appreciate. For now, we'll settle for a month in the Gulf Islands and Desolation if summer ever comes.

Besides, there's still a lot of you here in this house and we're not ready to just pack up. Speaking of which, your cremated remains are sitting here beside me. They don't come with an instruction manual either. We're thinking they belong in one or more of your favorite coves. But which ones? Maybe we'll stop by clinic and pick up a bunch of those urine specimen bottles that you liked and divide the ashes up into twenty or so bottles and have a bottle to scatter at each of your favorite places. One for Mexico too.

We're trying to adjust to life without fear. It's hard. I think we were fear junkies. Anyway, there are a lot of people who cared about you. Hundreds of cards. Emails. The Canucks sent a tree, and you've been in the local paper and the national television news. It's all been very nice. We're thinking about you and we miss you.

Dad

Cleaning Out the Dead Kid's Room

I think I'm supposed to share cute stories. You know the Thanksgiving stuff where I baked pies, but really only served as executive chef while Foster and his friends did the pastry and Tracey cooked the pumpkin filling. Or how rather than cooking Brussels sprouts, we launched them off Vicki's deck by slingshot into the sea forever confusing Yoshi on the tradition of Canadian Thanksgiving. Or I should talk about the paint ball and the bruises on my body or the smile on Foster's face. Or maybe tell tales of Tracey's training for the half marathon or Scupper's propensity to stop running and roll in dead salmon by the river bank and how good he smells after he's been washed in Foster's Axe because we're all out of doggie shampoo.

Maybe I should shockingly rip the tale in another direction and offer some poignant reminder that we are not just amazing people living life so fully, but newly wounded grieving folks able to triumph in the most difficult of circumstances.

Then you are supposed to go "wow" and have some moment of introspection wondering how we do it, and wonder if faced with similar circumstances, how would you react? How would you live your life? Maybe you can't answer the question. Maybe you are just glad you will never be faced with the question, touch wood.

Or perhaps I'm supposed to pull profound observations out of the air like, if we won a lottery, we would probably be packing up a boat and going for a nice long cruise in some tropical climate.

Conversely, if the economy sunk into a global depression and we lost our house and jobs, we would probably be packing up a boat and going for a nice long cruise in some tropical climate. The difference between the two is that in one case, fishing would be a recreational pursuit, and in the other, it would be a quest for protein to go with the rice and beans.

The two ends of the spectrum meet somewhere north of Panama or perhaps west of the Galapagos.

Which at this point should leave you wondering what the hell I'm talking about, and my clever obfuscation has left you thinking two levels deeper than I ever was. At this point, I would just end the story and you would feel good, or moved, or confused, and we would wait for the next one.

But it would all be a distortion because I never directly address the question about what it is like to be the father of a dead kid. And I can't possibly explain it. You nod your head with understanding and a large measure of pity, and I shake my head because you don't understand it. Because life is so fantastically ordinary. With work and report cards and dirty dog feet and obesity and soccer in the rain. The ordinary is wonderful and cherished, and my ordinary is at least twice as ordinary as yours. Except I cherish mine, which makes me extraordinary.

So never pity me or envy me. I couldn't give a damn if I ever win the lottery or if I am left homeless because either way, everything will still be okay, because we'll all be together. And I'll be fishing.

Oh, and Spence, I think about you every day, five months later. Love you, buddy.

Lo Siento, No Hablo Aburrido

I haven't written much lately. There were some good reasons why I was quiet. Some things were going on that I just wasn't at liberty to talk about, but now I am free.

Today, I was fired.

Nothing personal. Just one of those transactions where a business is bought and they didn't want all the bits of it so they get shut down and left behind. And so it was.

I wish I could say it was all very sad and tragic, which it is of course at one level, but at another level there is opportunity.

And so it is. My job is now to refit the boat and get the house ready, because the house will be rented, and the boat is going to Mexico.

Foster will be dragged from school. Now geography, biology, mathematics, social studies, physics, navigation, watch keeping, engine maintenance, and Spanish lessons will all happen in the cockpit and the salon of Blackdragon. A real education. Tracey gave notice at work today as well. We will leave in July or August, and we'll come back in time for school to start next year.

We couldn't be happier.

The planning is done. Now it's time to do something.

Crossing One Off the List

The income tax is filed. I have sewn a spinnaker for downwind sailing, complete with a snuffing sock.

The frames for the new bimini are installed, as is a new sub panel and mounting for the VHF radio, single sideband radio, and stereo. My fabric has arrived for me to sew the bimini top. Things are going well.

I crossed one other item off the list today.

The Gillette Series "Cool Cleansing" Shave Gel is intended for facial use only. Don't ask me why I know this.

Dr. Pollock was amazingly punctual. My appointment was for 10:10. At 10:25, I was standing in the lineup at Tim Horton's. Dr. Pollock's literature states that most men report no pain during the procedure.

Most men lie.

It might be "no needle", but having the anesthetic shot through your scrotum under high pressure isn't quite the same as a fairy sprinkling pixie dust. But it was all done in a few minutes. They asked if I experienced any pain.

I told them "No."

Again, I declined the deluxe post care pack. No need to pay $150 for a few dressings, a jock strap, some gel ice packs and a couple of Tylenol. Tracey had already taken care of it. Though she did buy frozen mixed vegetables instead of peas. It was quite a large bag. A little more thermal mass than I would have liked.

I had a day relaxing. I picked Foster up from school and prepared a simple dinner. I served grilled chicken with tortellini. I was just about to put the vegetables on Foster's plate and he said, "No thanks!"

"You have to have vegetables," I said.

"But I know where those have been."

I drove him to baseball, came back and watched the hockey game. Tracey picked him up from the game and they came home to find me relaxing on the couch with a smaller bag of vegetables. Foster wanted to know what the big deal was.

Tracey explained that I had a little cut on my scrotum.

"That's it? Just a little cut?" he mocked me.

I defended myself. "It wasn't just a little cut. There were stitches and a soldering iron and tubes pulled out and things."

"A soldering iron? Do you have metal balls?"

I liked him better when he was six. I could win then.

Birthday Greetings from the Sea of Cortez

Happy Birthday, Bud.

Thought I would drop you a line. I know I'm a day late, but hey, it's Mexico. We do the best we can.

We completely forgot Mother's Day this year. I blame it on Foster. He's the kid. It's called Mother's Day not Wife's Day, after all. Not really my problem. But we can't be too hard on him. After nearly a year on the boat, we are completely missing all the advertising and hoopla to ensure that we make the correct commercial choices to appropriately commemorate the occasion.

Thankfully, Mexico does it a day later so we were able to pretend that we just chose to celebrate it on Mexican time. Necklaces made with seashells we collect off the beach work fine. That, and dinner out for a change.

Sarah is with us. Her first day in the Sea of Cortez. Thanks for sending the two tuna. She enjoyed reeling them in. Oh yeah, and the manta rays. Hundreds of them. It was nice that they jumped right beside the boat too. We have video. And the dolphins. An anchorage full. You didn't have to send the big ones, but it was a nice touch.

Wow. Yet more days have passed since I started writing this. Now I'm really late. Sarah has been and gone and sends her love.

We never did catch a dorado or show her whales, but I think she had fun just the same.

We've been busting more stuff. Fried the alternator again and sheared the main shaft on the windlass. The new computer was destroyed in the chubasco and now I have a little netbook with a Spanish operating system and keyboard. So forgive the spelling mistakes. Oh yes, the outboard is dead. Connecting rod is severed and the bearings on the crankshaft are shot. I'm sure it's nothing that a thousand dollars' worth of Honda parts couldn't fix, if we could even get them here.

We've been trying to figure out how to get Blackdragon home and we may throw it on a ship that leaves La Paz on June 3. Then we just need to figure out how to get the other black dragon, El Scupper, back to Canada. It's hard to fly to Canada out of Mexico in the summertime because the airlines won't take dogs in the heat. Maybe we should put him in one of those little purses and tuck him under the seat in the cabin, or we may just rent cars and do the grand tour.

We're entering that phase where we wrap things up and start heading back to reality, whatever that is. Thanks for reminding us that reality is overrated and that life is really about living every day, sometimes simply, enjoying the scenery, the food, and the people you are with. And even if I only know eight notes on three strings, it still worth picking up the guitar and giving it a try. If only to stop Foster the mocker, who calls it a sitar because it spends all its time sitting on the shelf. But mostly because it feels good to make music.

So Spencer, we will be thinking about you tomorrow. I don't know what's more important, the day you were born or the day you died. Maybe neither. I think, perhaps, it was all the days that you lived.

We miss you.

Love,

Dad

Charities

A portion of the proceeds from the sale of this book will go towards the acquisition and provisioning of a sailboat with blue water capability and adequate rum storage; another portion will find its way to helping bald kids and their families. Consider making your gift of blood or money directly to some of our favourites:

Balding for Dollars

www.baldingfordollars.com

Children's Neuroblastoma Cancer Foundation

www.cncfhope.org

Solving Kids' Cancer

www.solvingkidscancer.org

The James Fund for Neuroblastoma Research

www.jamesfund.com

Children's Wish Foundation

www.childrenswish.ca

Canadian Blood Services

www.blood.ca

Printed in Canada